Health Informatics

This series is directed to healthcare professionals leading the transformation of healthcare by using information and knowledge. For over 20 years, Health Informatics has offered a broad range of titles: some address specific professions such as nursing, medicine, and health administration; others cover special areas of practice such as trauma and radiology; still other books in the series focus on interdisciplinary issues, such as the computer based patient record, electronic health records, and networked healthcare systems. Editors and authors, eminent experts in their fields, offer their accounts of innovations in health informatics. Increasingly, these accounts go beyond hardware and software to address the role of information in influencing the transformation of healthcare delivery systems around the world. The series also increasingly focuses on the users of the information and systems: the organizational, behavioral, and societal changes that accompany the diffusion of information technology in health services environments.

Developments in healthcare delivery are constant; in recent years, bioinformatics has emerged as a new field in health informatics to support emerging and ongoing developments in molecular biology. At the same time, further evolution of the field of health informatics is reflected in the introduction of concepts at the macro or health systems delivery level with major national initiatives related to electronic health records (EHR), data standards, and public health informatics.

These changes will continue to shape health services in the twenty-first century. By making full and creative use of the technology to tame data and to transform information, Health Informatics will foster the development and use of new knowledge in healthcare.

Peter L. Elkin
Editor

Terminology, Ontology and their Implementations

Teaching Guide and Notes

Springer

Editor
Peter L. Elkin
University at Buffalo, State University of New York
Buffalo, NY, USA

ISSN 1431-1917 ISSN 2197-3741 (electronic)
Health Informatics
ISBN 978-3-031-11301-7 ISBN 978-3-031-11302-4 (eBook)
https://doi.org/10.1007/978-3-031-11302-4

Spin-off ancillary Teachers manual providing extra detail building upon the content of: 87018565_ Elkin_Terminology, Ontology and their Implementations (978-3-031-11038-2)

This Springer imprint is published by the registered company Springer Nature Switzerland AG
The registered company address is: Gewerbestrasse 11, 6330 Cham, Switzerland

Springer Teachers' Guide

This teachers' guide is intended to supplement the Terminologies and Terminological Systems textbook. It provides answers and explanations for each of the questions at the back of the text. It also provides additional questions to be used in a final examination. It is organized by the chapter of the textbook and provides some of the goals of each chapter as an introduction to the questions and explanations.

Our goal is to be helpful to those teaching Health Informatics classes in their approach and development of curriculum for health terminologies and the systems needed for their development, dissemination, and implementation.

The actual questions follow are organized according to the sections of the textbook:

Theoretical Aspects of Ontology and Terminology

Preface

Questions

1. Which of the following is not a type of knowledge? (c)
   (a) Instance data
   (b) Ontological
   (c) Representational
   (d) Assertional
2. True or False, terminologies are used to populate mortality registries? True
3. What is the distinction between a controlled vocabulary and a terminology? (d)
   (a) A controlled vocabulary does not have concepts organized hierarchically
   (b) A terminology does not have concepts organized hierarchically
   (c) Controlled vocabularies are controlled by limiting what topics they can represent
   (d) They are synonymous
4. What is the goal of creating a controlled vocabulary? (b)
   (a) To keep your field from being easily understood by others
   (b) To aggregate information by meaning
   (c) To contain the assertional knowledge known by experts in the field
   (d) To keep track of specific patient's problems
5. A concept is unambiguous if it: (d)
   (a) Is able to be understood in two distinct ways
   (b) It has more than one meaning
   (c) If multiple readers can reasonably interpret the meaning of the concept differently
   (d) It has only one meaning

6. Which of the following pairs of concepts are redundant? (c)
   (a) Heart/Heart Attack
   (b) Myocardial Infarction/Acute Myocardial Infarction
   (c) Heart Muscle/Myocardium
   (d) Myocardial Infarction/Cardiovascular Disease
7. An example of a subtype hierarchy of concepts is: (d)
   (a) Entity/Disease/Cardiovascular Disease/Acute Myocardial Infarction/Myocardial Infarction
   (b) Acute Myocardial Infarction/Myocardial Infarction/Cardiovascular Disease/Disease/Entity
   (c) Disease/Cardiovascular Disease/Myocardial Infarction/Acute Myocardial Infarction/Entity
   (d) Entity/Disease/Cardiovascular Disease/Myocardial Infarction/Acute Myocardial Infarction
8. Systematic definitions are: (c)
   (a) Created by using terminological systems
   (b) Written by a computer
   (c) Follow a compositional method of defining the concepts
   (d) Follow rules for defining the identifiers associated with concepts
9. True or False, synonyms associated with concepts are given separate concept identifiers? False
10. Which of the following best describes the benefits of controlled terminologies? (d)
   (a) The aggregate information by meaning
   (b) They contain synonyms so that they can recognize multiple terms that represent the same concept or idea
   (c) They are arranged in hierarchies which allows users to get information stored that is related to a concept and all its children
   (d) All of the above

Buffalo, NY, USA — Peter L. Elkin
Buffalo, NY, USA — Barry Smith
Nashville, TN, USA — Steven H. Brown

Contents

Chapter 1
Introduction

Peter L. Elkin and Barry Smith

The introduction lays the foundation for the book. It presents a driving use case for terminologies and gives the reader some of the important definitions required to read and learn from the rest of the book. That said we have tried to let the chapters stand on their own recognizing that many Informatics courses may not cover the entire textbook.

P. L. Elkin (✉)
Department of Biomedical Informatics, Jacobs School of Medicine and Biomedical Sciences, University at Buffalo, State University of New York, Buffalo, NY, USA

Internal Medicine, Jacobs School of Medicine and Biomedical Sciences, University at Buffalo, State University of New York, Buffalo, NY, USA

Surgery, Jacobs School of Medicine and Biomedical Sciences, University at Buffalo, State University of New York, Buffalo, NY, USA

Pathology and Anatomical Sciences, Jacobs School of Medicine and Biomedical Sciences, University at Buffalo, State University of New York, Buffalo, NY, USA

Psychiatry, Jacobs School of Medicine and Biomedical Sciences, University at Buffalo, State University of New York, Buffalo, NY, USA

Orthopedics, Jacobs School of Medicine and Biomedical Sciences, University at Buffalo, State University of New York, Buffalo, NY, USA
e-mail: elkinp@buffalo.edu;
http://medicine.buffalo.edu/departments/biomedical-informatics.html

B. Smith
Department of Philosophy, University at Buffalo, Buffalo, NY, USA

Department of Biomedical Informatics, University at Buffalo, Buffalo, NY, USA
e-mail: phismith@buffalo.edu

P. L. Elkin (ed.), *Terminology, Ontology and their Implementations*, Health Informatics, https://doi.org/10.1007/978-3-031-11302-4_1

Questions

1. Which of the following is not a type of knowledge? (c)

   (a) Instance data
   (b) Ontological
   (c) Representational
   (d) Assertional

   The three types of knowledge are Ontological (i.e., definitional knowledge), Assertional knowledge (or facts about in this use case health and healthcare) and Instance data (the assignment of knowledge to an individual or situation). Therefore, the correct answer is (c) that Representational knowledge is not a primary knowledge type.
2. True or False, terminologies are used to populate Mortality registries? True

   Terminological data is used for both mortality and morbidity coding. Terminologies may be constructed to better serve one of these goals.
3. What is the distinction between a controlled vocabulary and a terminology? (d)

   (a) A controlled vocabulary does not have concepts organized hierarchically
   (b) A terminology does not have concepts organized hierarchically
   (c) Controlled vocabularies are controlled by limiting what topics they can represent
   (d) They are synonymous

   Authors in Health Informatics have at times developed in this author's opinion hair splitting distinctions between a controlled vocabulary and a terminology. These distinctions have been used inconsistently across the literature and since the degree of inter-rater reliability of these names is low, for the purposes of this textbook, we define a terminology to be a controlled vocabulary. Also we define a controlled vocabulary to be a terminology, that is to say they are synonymous concepts.
4. What is the goal of creating a controlled vocabulary? (b)

   (a) To keep your field from being easily understood by others
   (b) To aggregate information by meaning
   (c) To contain the assertional knowledge known by experts in the field
   (d) To keep track of specific patient's problems

   Terminology used in any technical field can be both an aid and a barrier to understanding. Simply put the idea of any controlled vocabulary is to fix the meaning of a concept and to aggregate data at the level of that meaning. This allows reproducible and credible tagging of information that can later be understood to have the same meaning as the recorder intended.
5. A concept is unambiguous if it: (d)

   (a) Is able to be understood in two distinct ways
   (b) It has more than one meaning

(c) If multiple readers can reasonably interpret the meaning of the concept differently
(d) It has only one meaning

A concept is unambiguous if it has only one meaning. Said another way, no concept can have more than one meaning. This is necessary for there to be a high level of inter-rater agreement when reading stored data.

6. Which of the following pairs of concepts are redundant? (c)

(a) Heart/heart attack
(b) Myocardial infarction/acute myocardial infarction
(c) Heart muscle/myocardium
(d) Myocardial infarction/cardiovascular disease

A redundant concept is where two concepts, identified by different codes (identifiers), have the same meaning. In this case, *Heart Muscle* and *Myocardium* are synonyms and therefore have the same meaning. If they were to have different identifiers, they would be redundant concepts. *Heart* and *Heart Attack* are different concepts (although *Heart Attack* can be defined in part by HasFindingsite *Heart*). *Acute Myocardial Infarction* is a subtype of *Myocardial Infarction* which is a subtype of *Cardiovascular Disease*.

7. An example of a subtype hierarchy of concepts is: (d)

(a) Entity/disease/cardiovascular disease/acute myocardial infarction/myocardial infarction
(b) Acute myocardial infarction/myocardial infarction/cardiovascular disease/disease/entity
(c) Disease/cardiovascular disease/myocardial infarction/acute myocardial infarction/entity
(d) Entity/disease/cardiovascular disease/myocardial infarction/acute myocardial infarction

Only item (d) has a hierarchy that goes consistently from more general to more specific. In (a), *Acute Myocardial infarction* should not come before *Myocardial Infarction*. In (b), the hierarchy is from more specific to more general. In (c), the concept *entity* is the most general not the most specific concept.

8. Systematic definitions are: (c)

(a) Created by using terminological systems
(b) Written by a computer
(c) Follow a compositional method of defining the concepts
(d) Follow rules for defining the identifiers associated with concepts

Systematic definitions require one to know if any definable part of the concept has already received a definition. When the answer to that question is yes, then the definition for the part of the concept needs to be incorporated exactly into the definition of its more complex-related concept. For example, if we have a definition of *Infarction* and we want to define a *Myocardial Infarction*, the systematic definition for *Myocardial Infarction* would necessarily include the definition for *Infarction*. This is important as a *Myocardial Infarction* is an *Infarction* and therefore would inherit the properties of an *Infarction*.

9. True or False synonyms associated with concepts are given separate concept identifiers? (a)

   (a) False
   (b) True

   This is clearly false. Synonyms, by definition, have the same meaning. If a synonym was given a separate identifier in the terminology, this would lead to ambiguous representations. If both concepts were utilized to record data, information retrieval using either of the two concepts would then return less than the full amount of data for any given query without this being easily known to the investigator.

10. Which of the following best describes the benefits of controlled terminologies? (d)

    (a) The aggregate information by meaning
    (b) They contain synonymy so that they can recognize multiple terms that represent the same concept or idea
    (c) They are arranged in hierarchies which allows users to get information stored that is related to a concept and all its children
    (d) All of the above

    The benefits of the use of a controlled terminology include aggregation of data by its meaning. Terminologies also provide the ability to recognize multiple surface forms (synonymous terms) which convey the meaning of the concept. The hierarchical arrangement of concepts contains information that allows a user to query all the concepts in the tree by choosing only the top node needed. This leads to efficiencies in data aggregation and in the use of terminologies for information retrieval.

Chapter 2
History of Terminology

Peter L. Elkin and Barry Smith

The history of terminology is a broad field. In this chapter, we have tried to highlight the contributions of just a few of the many individuals over the last almost 2.4 Millenia that have contributed to our knowledge of terminologies as controlled representations with particular attention to their application in health and healthcare. We take the field along with its illustrious champions from an observational to a logical science. In this way, we link domain knowledge with the scientific method and a set of formal mathematics for knowledge representation. This moves our field from a descriptive to a computer science in the field of Health Informatics.

P. L. Elkin (✉)
Department of Biomedical Informatics, Jacobs School of Medicine and Biomedical Sciences, University at Buffalo, State University of New York, Buffalo, NY, USA

Internal Medicine, Jacobs School of Medicine and Biomedical Sciences, University at Buffalo, State University of New York, Buffalo, NY, USA

Surgery, Jacobs School of Medicine and Biomedical Sciences, University at Buffalo, State University of New York, Buffalo, NY, USA

Pathology and Anatomical Sciences, Jacobs School of Medicine and Biomedical Sciences, University at Buffalo, State University of New York, Buffalo, NY, USA

Psychiatry, Jacobs School of Medicine and Biomedical Sciences, University at Buffalo, State University of New York, Buffalo, NY, USA

Orthopedics, Jacobs School of Medicine and Biomedical Sciences, University at Buffalo, State University of New York, Buffalo, NY, USA
e-mail: elkinp@buffalo.edu;
http://medicine.buffalo.edu/departments/biomedical-informatics.html

B. Smith
Department of Philosophy, University at Buffalo, Buffalo, NY, USA

Department of Biomedical Informatics, University at Buffalo, Buffalo, NY, USA
e-mail: phismith@buffalo.edu

P. L. Elkin (ed.), *Terminology, Ontology and their Implementations*, Health Informatics, https://doi.org/10.1007/978-3-031-11302-4_2

Our history starts with Hippocrates and progresses to the work of Aristotle. The advent of the Guttenberg printing press showed a great expansion of knowledge dissemination and the need for better indexing and classification. As we moved through the renaissance to the industrial revolution, we see science and formal logics replacing or more appropriately expanding our logical basis for knowledge representation. Charles Morris and Pierce bring in a new age of logical definitions which expand our understanding and form the basis for systematic definitions and more modern terminologies. With modern computing iterative solutions became possible and logical formalisms that require recursive reasoning found their place in our lexicon. As we move further into the twenty-first century, we have a rich set of semantic tools with which to craft and utilize the knowledge available in our compositional terminologies.

Questions

1. Who developed the first health-related terminology? (d)

   (a) Heraclides
   (b) Aristotle
   (c) Plato
   (d) Hippocrates

   Although Aristotle may have created the first logical terminologies for science, Hippocrates created the first health-related terminologies at least 100 years earlier. His Corpus of Hippocrates held classifications for organ system-based disease and types of surgical procedures. Heraclides was Hippocrates's father and Plato was Aristotle's professor but was not senior to Hippocrates.

2. Who is the father of modern medical statistics? (b)

   (a) Aristotle
   (b) William Farr
   (c) Charles Peirce
   (d) Adolphe Quetelet

   William Farr was a British epidemiologist who was the president of the royal statistical society and formed the first catalog of vital statistics which held causes of death by occupation. Peirce was a logician and Quetelet was a nineteenth century social statistician. Aristotle to our knowledge did not compile death registries.

3. All are examples of Universals except? (d)

   (a) A tree
   (b) Good
   (c) Evil
   (d) Mount Fuji

   Aristotle's principle of Universals and Instances defined the idea of a concept as the universal and the instance as the particular. An example of a universal is the abstract concept of a tree. This could be any tree of any type, of any age and in any location. The particular of a tree would be a specific tree. Associated with that tree would be its specific species, age, and location. Aristotle's idea of universality extended to conceptual notions such as good or evil. These exist and can be defined but are not instances of an evil act for example. In this list, the only specific entity is Mount Fuji which is a specific mountain rather than the abstract concept of a mountain.

4. Which concept would be considered a particular? (a)

   (a) Gone with the Wind
   (b) A Mountain
   (c) Happiness
   (d) Pain

   A particular is an instance in the real world. In this case, Gone with the Wind is a specific book or movie rather than the abstract concept of a book or a movie. Unlike Universals they identify real-world-specific objects or entities. A mountain is an abstract concept as is Happiness or Pain, and therefore they are universals and not particulars as represented by Aristotle.

5. Aristotle's E-type is exemplified by: (d)

   (a) A person with blond hair
   (b) All people are born with blue eyes
   (c) All cars have an engine
   (d) All people are not on Mars

   Aristotle's E-type is universal and negative such as "No one is immortal." Immortal is negative, so answer (d) "All people are not on Mars" is the correct response. Here all people are a Universal and not on Mars is a negative making this an E-type proposition. A person with blond hair is an I-type which is particular and positive. All people are born with blue eyes is universal and affirmative and therefore is of Aristotle type A. All cars have an engine is also a type A Aristotle proposition.

6. Aristotle's O-type is exemplified by: (b)

   (a) Some people have blue eyes
   (b) Some people don't like chocolate ice cream
   (c) Some people run to stay in shape
   (d) All of the above

   Aristotle's O-type propositions are particular and negative. All of these responses are particular and the only item with a negative premise is item (b) which states that some people don't like chocolate ice cream. Therefore, items (a) and (c) are particulars and affirmative making them Aristotle I-type expressions. All of the above is incorrect as (a) and (c) are incorrect.

7. The precursor of the International Classification of Diseases was? (a)

   (a) The London Bills of Mortality
   (b) The Organon

(c) The US Classification of Diseases
(d) The French Classification of Diseases

The London Bills of mortality developed in the mid-nineteenth century was very successful and paved the way for the development of the International Classification of Diseases which are now maintained by the World Health Organization. The Organon was the grammar and rules for the construction of the language of logic written by Aristotle.

8. Semantics are? (d)

(a) The form of an expression
(b) The terms in an expression
(c) The concepts in an expression
(d) The meaning of an expression

Expressions are made up of both content and semantics. The content defines the thoughts that are represented and the semantics define the meaning of the expression. The semantics contain logic, often description logic defining exactly the meaning of the expression. The form of the expression is its syntax. The terms in an expression are the surface forms used to represent the concepts in a human readable form, and the concepts are the entities and ideas used in the expression. Although concepts carry meaning, the semantics of an expression, whether pre-coordinated or post-coordinated, requires a grammar and a set of logics to link sets of concepts into one or more compositional expressions.

9. Semantics can be represented as: (d)

(a) A set of propositions
(b) Concept and relationship/concept triples
(c) A syllogism
(d) All of the above

A set of propositions or a set of concept triples with two concepts linked by a relationship are semantic representations of information. A syllogism is a proposition which follows from two or more other propositions. This is also called by some authors a logical argument or a simple proof. All of these statements are semantic representations, therefore the correct response is (d).

10. Logical positivism was applied to: (c)

(a) Science and biology
(b) Biology and psychology
(c) Psychology and science
(d) Science and biology

Logical positivism was defined in the book *Principia Mathematica* published by Russell and Whitehead in the 1920s and showed that mathematics as indeed logical. This principle of logical positivism was subsequently applied to the fields of psychology and science.

Chapter 3
Theoretical Foundations of Terminology

Peter L. Elkin and Steven H. Brown

The Theoretical Foundations of Terminology reflect the basic principles of what indicates quality in a terminology and how to rate interoperability provided by a terminological standard or implementation or system. These basic notions are the cornerstone of understanding that one needs to select, make use of or design terminologies or terminological systems. We begin by discussing the various types of terminologies and move to best practices of terminology development and use and then close with a discussion of interoperability where we present a validated scale for the measurement of the level of interoperability provided by any specific terminological standard

P. L. Elkin (✉)
Department of Biomedical Informatics, Jacobs School of Medicine and Biomedical Sciences, University at Buffalo, State University of New York, Buffalo, NY, USA

Internal Medicine, Jacobs School of Medicine and Biomedical Sciences, University at Buffalo, State University of New York, Buffalo, NY, USA

Surgery, Jacobs School of Medicine and Biomedical Sciences, University at Buffalo, State University of New York, Buffalo, NY, USA

Pathology and Anatomical Sciences, Jacobs School of Medicine and Biomedical Sciences, University at Buffalo, State University of New York, Buffalo, NY, USA

Psychiatry, Jacobs School of Medicine and Biomedical Sciences, University at Buffalo, State University of New York, Buffalo, NY, USA

Orthopedics, Jacobs School of Medicine and Biomedical Sciences, University at Buffalo, State University of New York, Buffalo, NY, USA
e-mail: elkinp@buffalo.edu;
http://medicine.buffalo.edu/departments/biomedical-informatics.html

S. H. Brown
Department of Veterans Affairs, Office of Health Informatics, Knowledge Based Systems, Washington, DC, USA

Department of Biomedical Informatics, Vanderbilt University, Nashville, TN, USA
e-mail: steven.brown@va.gov

P. L. Elkin (ed.), *Terminology, Ontology and their Implementations*, Health Informatics, https://doi.org/10.1007/978-3-031-11302-4_3

or implementation or system. These fundamentals will assist the reader in the proper interpretation of the chapters which follow this one in the textbook.

Questions

1. The simplest form of hierarchies are? (b)

   (a) Ordinal lists
   (b) Lists within lists
   (c) Groups of lists
   (d) Non-ordinal lists

   Categorized lists are the simplest form of terminology. The simplest form of terminological hierarchy are lists within lists and therefore (b) is the correct item. Ordinal lists are ordered lists, groups of lists need not be related and non-ordinal lists are lists that are unordered, none of which necessarily meet the criteria for a hierarchically arranged terminology.

2. A canonical term in a terminology is? (c)

   (a) The first term in the terminology
   (b) The last term in the terminology
   (c) The preferred term for a concept
   (d) A synonym of the preferred term for a concept

   A canonical term is the preferred term for a concept (answer (c)) within a specific version of a terminology. Synonyms are other equivalent surface forms of the concept that can include traditional synonyms, acronyms and abbreviations. The first and last terms in the terminology are not necessarily canonical terms.

3. Concept orientation of a terminology means? (a)

   (a) That the concept is the basic organization of meaning
   (b) The concept is an abstract notion
   (c) The concept orientation is a hierarchy within the terminology
   (d) The concept identifier is the meaning of the concept

   For a terminology to be concept oriented, the meaning of the terminology should be organized around the concept. Best practice reflects that this is organized around a meaningless identifier which is logically connected to both a systematic and formal definition of the concept. Canonical and synonymous terms associated with the concept may be in multiple languages and have a variety of encoding formats (e.g. ASCII, UTF-8). Although context within a terminology is important for consistency and meaning, neither the hierarchical placement of the concept nor its identifier impart the entire definition or meaning to the concept. The abstract notion of a concept applies to all concepts but does not define a specific concept.

4. Vagueness in a terminology occurs when? (d)

   (a) A term is not well written
   (b) A concept is not well written

(c) There is more than one concept with the same meaning
(d) The concept is context dependent
(e) There is more than one meaning for a concept

Concepts in a terminology should retain their meaning independent of context. If we have a hierarchy and a subtype of the concept *Diabetes Mellitus* is *Type I*, then the meaning of *Type I* which in this case is *Type I Diabetes Mellitus* is only retained while the hierarchical connection to *Diabetes Mellitus* is retained. Best practice in terminological development would expect the hierarchy to have a term *Diabetes Mellitus* and a subtype of *Type I Diabetes Mellitus*. This later example would not be vague and would meet a higher standard of terminological development. Answer (c) is an example of redundancy and answer (e) is an example of ambiguity.

5. Redundancy happens when? (c)

(a) A term is not well written
(b) A concept is not well written
(c) There is more than one concept with the same meaning
(d) The concept is context free
(e) There is more than one meaning for a concept

By definition, redundancy occurs when the terminology has more than one concept, each with separate identifiers, which have the same meaning. Answer (e) is an example of ambiguity.

6. Ambiguity happens in a terminology when? (e)

(a) A term is not well written
(b) A concept is not well written
(c) There is more than one concept with the same meaning
(d) The concept is context free
(e) There is more than one meaning for a concept

Ambiguity occurs when there is more than one meaning for a single concept within a terminology. Answer (c) is the definition of redundancy and (d) is the definition of non-vagueness.

7. Internal consistency within a terminology means that? (a)

(a) Relationships between concepts should be uniform across parallel domains within the terminology
(b) Relationships follow the Isa relation
(c) Relationships follow the part of relation
(d) Relationships between concepts should be uniform within parallel domains across the terminology

For a terminology to be consistent, any relationship between a concept and its subtypes for example should be the same regardless of from which hierarchy one reaches that concept. Internal consistency also requires that the application of relationships uses the same definition for the relation regardless of the subdomain being addressed. For example, the HasMorphology relation from SNOMED CT should have the same meaning and application in Cardiology as in Gastroenterology. Also required by this concept of internal consistency is that the relation be applied everywhere in the terminology that it would make sense to apply that relationship. This leads to the consistent application of the relation. Answer (d) is within hierarchies or domains and that makes (a) the superior response for this question.

8. The content coverage of the terminology =? (c)

   (a) The number of concepts in the terminology that cover concepts from the real world/The number of concepts in the real world
   (b) The number of domain concepts in the terminology that cover concepts from the real world/The number of concepts in the real world
   (c) The number of domain concepts in the terminology that cover concepts from the same domain from the real world/The number of concepts in the domain within the real world
   (d) The number of concepts in the domain of the real world/The number of concepts in the terminology

   The content coverage of the terminology relates the content of the terminology to the content in the domain that is the scope of the terminology in the real world. This is usually determined by comparing the terminology against live data from the domain. Here the right equation is the number of domain concepts from the terminology divided by the number of domain concepts within the real world. With this measure we are not determining whether the terminology has the surface forms (terms) to represent the exact string, but rather whether the meaning associated with the term found in the real world is covered by the content of the terminology. Answer (a) and (b) are incorrect as it does not limit the real-world concepts to the domain in scope. Answer (d) does not make sense.

9. Mapping between terminologies is accomplished by? (a)

   (a) Mapping the meaning of concepts of the two terminologies
   (b) Mapping the terms of the two terminologies
   (c) Mapping the hierarchies of the two terminologies
   (d) Mapping the relationships of the two terminologies

   The key point to this question is that mapping exercises are about meaning and not surface forms (lexical elements). The meaning is determined by context (relationships) as well as definitions. When mapping two pre-coordinated terminologies, our group has found in the domain of diagnoses that there is for ICD9-CM and other diagnostic terminologies only a 33% lexical match rate, however by mapping two pre-coordinated terminologies to SNOMED CT and matching across SNOMED CT concepts associated with the pre-coordinations we were able to match up to 95% of the terms in the two diagnostic terminologies. Answers (b), (c) and (d) are incorrect as they are each alone insufficient criteria for the creation of accurate mappings.

10. A composite concept is? (d)

    (a) Any pre-coordinated concept
    (b) Any post-coordinated concept
    (c) Any concept with a formal definition
    (d) Any pre- or post-coordinated concept

    Composite concepts are synonymous with non-atomic concepts. Atomic concepts are concepts that cannot be further divided into two or more elements and retain its meaning. So if we could create a compositional structure from the terminological elements to create the concept is by definition a composite concept. These are pre-coordinated if they exist with a unique identifier within the terminology, and they are post-coordinated if they do not exist in the terminology but can be constructed by creating a compositional expression made up of concepts and relationships limited to those found in the same terminology. Answer (b) is true but insufficient to define the set of composite concepts. Answers (a) and (c) are equivalent for a compositional terminology but are again insufficient as they exclude post-coordinations.
11. Atomic concepts are? (b)

    (a) Concepts that are made up of atoms
    (b) Concepts that cannot be further decomposed in the terminology
    (c) Concepts that have been used in pre-coordinated concepts
    (d) Concepts that have been used in post-coordinated concepts

    Atomic concepts are those that cannot be further decomposed in a specific terminology. These can be used in the construction of pre- or post-coordinated concepts; however, this is not a requirement for their status as an atomic concept therefore answers (c) and (d) are incorrect. Answer (a) is the incorrect as concepts that are made up of atoms can be further decomposed into those atoms.
12. Concept is to be termed as? (c)

    (a) Watermelon is to seed
    (b) House is to furniture
    (c) Idea is to name
    (d) Thought is to being

    This is an analogy problem. Concept is the idea and term is the name, therefore, (c) is the correct answer. House is to furniture describes what is contained in a house. A seed is contained in or used to grow a watermelon. Thought is to being is an existential concept that does not relate to the identification or labelling of a concept.
13. A synonym is an? (d)

    (a) Abbreviation
    (b) Acronym
    (c) Homonym
    (d) a and b
    (e) a, b and c

Types of synonyms include abbreviations and acronyms. Homonyms are words with the same pronunciation but based on their context can have different meanings. Therefore (d) is the correct answer.

14. Pre-coordinated concepts are? (b)

    (a) Those concepts that are created before the terminology is created
    (b) Those concepts that can be defined by more than one concept in the terminology
    (c) Those concepts that are created before the terminology is coordinated
    (d) Those concepts that are created before the terminology is finalized

    The definition of a pre-coordinated concept is that it can be fully defined by two or more concepts from the same terminology each pair being linked by a relationship. Therefore (b) is the correct answer. Answer (a) is incorrect as atomic concepts are also created when the terminology is constructed. Answers (c) and (d) are also too general and do not provide a definition of pre-coordination.

15. Post-coordinated concepts are? (a)

    (a) Those that are created from multiple concepts in the terminology and that do not themselves exist as concepts within the terminology
    (b) Those that are created from multiple concepts in the terminology that do themselves exist as concepts within the terminology
    (c) Those that are created from multiple concepts in the terminology and joined with concepts outside the terminology
    (d) Those that are created from multiple concepts in the terminology and then mapped to other terminologies

    Post-coordinations are made up of concepts in the terminology but create concepts that do not exist in the terminology as either atomic or pre-coordinated concepts. If as in (b) they do exist, then they would be pre-coordinations. The important point is that pre-coordinations are part of the terminology and shipped with the terminology, whereas post-coordinations are generally constructed at run time by end users who are trying to represent a meaning not contained in the terminology but which through logic can be constructed. Neither pre- or post-coordinations use concepts from outside of the terminology, therefore answers (c) and (d) are not correct.

16. A Kernel concept is? (c)

    (a) A concept that is at the centre of the terminology
    (b) A concept that represents the main meaning of a pre-coordinated concept
    (c) A concept that represents the main meaning of a pre- or post-coordinated concept
    (d) A concept that represents the main meaning of a post-coordinated concept

    Kernel concepts are concepts which can be the main idea of a compositional expression. These can be atomic concepts or pre-coordinations. However, we only need to make this distinction in the context of how the concepts are to be used in compositional expressions or how they are to be parsed by natural language processing systems. The Kernel concepts have no relationship to their hierarchical position in the terminology and as the meaning extends to both pre- and post-coordinated concepts, answers (c) and (d) are incorrect.

17. A modifier is? (a)

    (a) A concept that modifies the meaning of coordinated concept in a clinical sense
    (b) A concept that modifies the meaning of pre-coordinated concept in a clinical sense
    (c) A concept that modifies the meaning of post-coordinated concept in a clinical sense
    (d) A concept that modifies the meaning of an atomic concept in a clinical sense

    A modifier we have defined as a concept that modifies the meaning of a pre- or post-coordinated concept in a clinical sense. Therefore (a) is the correct answer. Atomic concepts do not contain modifiers. Primitive concepts and atomic concepts are synonyms as used in this textbook. Answers (b) and (c) do not either cover both pre- and post-coordinated concepts.

18. A qualifier is? (a)

    (a) A concept that modifies the meaning of coordinated concept in a temporal or administrative sense
    (b) A concept that modifies the meaning of pre-coordinated concept in a temporal or administrative sense
    (c) A concept that modifies the meaning of post-coordinated concept in a temporal or administrative sense
    (d) A concept that modifies the meaning of an atomic concept in a temporal or administrative sense

    A qualifier is a concept that modifies the meaning of a pre- or post-coordinated concept in a temporal or administrative sense. This includes concepts such as *before*, *during* or *after* and *status-post*, concepts such as *history of* or *family history of* would also be included. These combine more reliably into compositional expressions. Based on this the correct answer is (a).

19. Consistency of view means that? (d)

    (a) The interface to the terminology should not change between terminologies
    (b) The direction of the hierarchies should not change within a terminology
    (c) The meaning of a terminology should not change over time
    (d) The concepts should have the same descendants regardless of their parentage

    Consistency of view expresses the notion that the meaning of a concept is defined by its relationships. As there are multiple ways to get to the same concept moving down the hierarchy, meaning that the terminology can be polyhierarchical. For example, *Colon Cancer* can be both a *GI Disorder* and a *Malignant Neoplasm*. Consistency of view means that regardless of whether come to the concept *Colon Cancer* from *GI Disorders* or as a *Malignant Neoplasm* it has the same relationships and formal definition.

20. Explicitness of relations means that? (b)

    (a) Relations should have the same meaning throughout the terminology
    (b) Relations should have the same meaning and be used consistently throughout the terminology
    (c) Relations should be used consistently throughout the terminology
    (d) Relations should only change their meaning under specific circumstances within a terminology

    The notion of the explicitness of relations is that relationships should have the same meaning and be used consistently throughout the terminology. This means that the relations are applied in the same fashion and applied to all of the concepts that meet the class criteria for either the Operand or the Specification for the relationship. For example, HasEtiology might have the form *Infectious Disorder* HasEtiology *Organism*. This is not to imply that all organisms can cause all infectious disorders but to say that this is a legal relationship and that all such relations should be tested for their appropriateness for modelling.

21. A rule that governs the sign of concepts is? (c)

    (a) Concept orientation
    (b) Non-redundancy
    (c) Explicit uncertainty
    (d) Non-vagueness
    (e) Non-ambiguity

    The sign of a concept is its associated multi-valued logic truth value. For example, assertions associated with negative truth values are equivalent to zero (on a normalized scale of 0–1). Whereas assertions that are true are associated with a truth value of 1. A concept that is just as likely true as false would have a truth value of 0.5 on this normalized scale. Previous research has shown good inter-rater reliability for the following values:

    True—1.0
    Almost certainly true—0.951 → 0.999
    More likely true than false—0.51 → 0.95
    Just as likely true as false—0.5
    More likely false than true—0.499 → 0.05
    Almost certainly false—0.049 → 0.001
    False—0

    The principle of explicitness of uncertainty reflects the need to specify exactly the level of confidence of any assertion. Concept orientation relates to how meaning is organized in the terminology. Non-redundancy is the principle stating that no two concepts should have the same meaning. Non-vagueness is the principle stating that all concepts should retain their meaning outside of their hierarchical context. Non-ambiguity is the principle that no concept should have more than one meaning.

22. Normalization of content is? (a)

    (a) The process of supporting and mapping alternative words and shorthand terms for composite concepts
    (b) The process of mapping concepts from one terminology to another terminology
    (c) The process of mapping the semantics of one terminology to another terminology
    (d) The process or recognizing all ways that the semantics can be used to represent the same meaning

    Normalization of content is the process of supporting and mapping alternative words and shorthand terms for composite concepts. This in combination with semantic normalization ensures that there is no unrecognized ambiguity in the terminology. This relates to clinical understanding. If there are terms that have a clinical meaning that overlap this fact should be recognized and accounted for within the relationships contained within the terminology. All of the normalization is within the same terminology so answers (b) and (c) are incorrect. Answer (d) is the definition of semantic normalization.
23. Semantic normalization is? (d)

    (a) The process of supporting and mapping alternative words and shorthand terms for composite concepts
    (b) The process of mapping concepts from one terminology to another terminology
    (c) The process of mapping the semantics of one terminology to another terminology
    (d) The process or recognizing all ways that the semantics can be used to represent the same meaning

    Semantic normalization is the process or recognizing all ways that the semantics can be used to represent the same meaning (answer (d)). The answer (a) is the definition of content normalization. All of the normalization is within the same terminology so answers (b) and (c) are incorrect.
24. Context-free identifier are? (b)

    (a) An unbinding of the concept and the identifier
    (b) Concept identifiers whose format does not carry meaning
    (c) An unbinding of the concept from the terminology
    (d) Concept identifiers that do not associate with concepts that carry meaning

    A context-free identifier is the form of an identifier for the concepts in a terminology whose format does not carry meaning. There are many terminologies where the concept IDs are sequential. This can lead to a situation where you literally run out of room in an area of the hierarchy. With meaningless identifiers this cannot happen. Additionally meaningless identifiers do not need to be changed as the definition of the concept is updated which may cause trouble with stored data in the case of meaningful identifiers. The unbinding of concepts (b) and (c) could change the meaning of stored data and the last answer (d) is nonsensical.

25. Persistence of identifiers means? (c)

    (a) That identifiers are only reused when the concept is deleted
    (b) That identifiers are deleted when the concept is deleted
    (c) That the identifiers are never deleted
    (d) That the identifiers are always reused

    The persistence of identifiers means that identifiers are never deleted. If they are no longer valid, they are marked as obsolete. If there exists a new concept that better expresses the idea, then there is a pointer to that new concept from the old one. We had a good example of this notion that occurred some years ago when we originally thought that the virus that led to AIDS was the HTLV III virus. When we discovered that HIV virus was the virus that truly caused AIDS, we marked the first concept as obsolete and pointed it to the new concept of HIV. As identifiers are never deleted answers (a) and (b) are incorrect. Identifiers are never reused as this could lead to a change in meaning for data already stored in patients' clinical records.
26. Obsolescence marking is exemplified by? (d)

    (a) Marking a concept that is old
    (b) Marking a concept that is deleted
    (c) Marking a concept whose surface form has changed its meaning
    (d) Marking a concept that has been deleted or whose surface form has changed its meaning

    Obsolescence marking is a concept that has been deleted or whose surface form has changed its meaning. A concept can be old and not obsolete. Answers (b) and (c) are both only part of the answer whereas (d) presents the complete answer.
27. Obsolescence marking requires? (b)

    (a) Just the marking of the concept
    (b) Marking the concept and pointing to the new concept with the modified meaning
    (c) Marking the concept and showing its age
    (d) Marking its age and showing all the concepts with that age

    Obsolescence marking requires "marking" the concept and pointing to the new concept with the modified meaning. It is important to both mark the concept and also to create a pointer to the new updated concept as it is important when aggregating data to be able to include all relevant data. Often this occurs when we learn more about a disease and therefore need to update our definitions. However when aggregating data from patient records we may want to include data before and after the change was implemented.
28. Language independence for a terminology means? (a)

    (a) That it supports multiple languages
    (b) That it does not need a language to represent its knowledge

(c) That it has a concept identifier
(d) That it mixes multiple languages as synonyms

Language independence for a terminology means that it supports multiple languages. Although answers (b), (c) and (d) are all true, they are not the definition of language independence.

29. Precision is? (a)

(a) The true positive over the true positive plus the false-positive rates
(b) The true positive over the true positive plus the false-negative rates
(c) The true negative over the true positive plus the false-positive rates
(d) The true negative over the true positive plus the false-negative rates

This is a statistical definition. Precision is equivalent to the positive predictive value. Therefore, the precision is the true-positive rate divided by the true positives plus the false positives.

30. Recall is? (b)

(a) The true positive over the true positive plus the false-positive rates
(b) The true positive over the true positive plus the false-negative rates
(c) The true negative over the true positive plus the false-positive rates
(d) The true negative over the true positive plus the false-negative rates

Recall is used in information retrieval and is equivalent to sensitivity. Therefore, the recall is the true-positive rate divided by the true positives plus the false negatives.

31. Assertional knowledge is/are? (c)

(a) Ontological knowledge
(b) Facts about the terminology
(c) Facts about the domain expressed in the terminology
(d) Axioms defining the terminology

Assertional knowledge in healthcare are non-definitional facts within the domain of healthcare. These facts can be expressed using concepts from a terminology. These can be exemplified by facts such as "A flail mitral leaflet can lead to flash pulmonary edema." This makes item (c) the correct answer which reflects that this type of knowledge represents facts about a domain not about the terminology itself. We use axioms to represent the knowledge but those that define the terminology are specifically excluded therefore item (d) is incorrect. Ontological knowledge is definitional so this is also incorrect as is facts about terminology which are definitional.

32. Usability testing is appropriate? (d)

(a) When you can find typical participants
(b) When you are willing to make changes to the system
(c) When you run at least six participants through a set of structured scenarios
(d) All of the above

In order to have a valid usability test, you need to find typical participants for the study and run at least six participants through a set of structured scenarios. Also, it is not useful to perform a usability study unless you are willing to make changes to the system based on what you learn. Conversely, if you are not willing to make changes to the system there is really no point in running a usability study. Answer (d) all of the above is correct.

33. Usability testing should be performed? (d)

    (a) As soon as you think of a system design
    (b) As soon as you have a design specification to test
    (c) As soon as you have a version of the system ready for Beta testing
    (d) As you need information to make design choices throughout the development lifecycle

    You should consider undergoing usability testing as you need information to make design choices throughout the development lifecycle. There is no specific time in the software quality assurance lifecycle where you must do usability testing. The decision to test should be driven by the need for information that will help to improve the development or implementation or maintenance of the system. Therefore, (d) is the correct answer.

34. Steps in running a usability experiment include all except? (b)

    (a) Cognitive task analysis
    (b) Specifying a new system design based on the usability data
    (c) Developing typical scenarios for the study
    (d) Recruiting typical participants for the study

    Usability testing can include cognitive task analysis to determine which scenarios are best to test in the experiment. The participants and scenarios used in the study should reflect the personnel and workflows that will be used in practice. You would not specify a new system design based on a usability study as the functionality of the system is often separate from its usability.

35. All of these are potentially useful usability results except? (a)

    (a) Making leadership aware of the good work performed by the development team
    (b) Making the development team aware of usability errors
    (c) Making the development team aware of design elements that worked well
    (d) Making the usability team and the design team aware of issues for further usability studies

    Usability laboratories cost money to build. They are nice/interesting spaces within an organization. People associated with usability laboratories often want credit for their good work. Sometimes this leads to the misuse of the lab in terms of using leadership as study participants to make them aware of the lab and its good work. This can lead to altered study results that can mislead the development team leading to unusable systems. The other answers are correct. Usability studies are designed to inform the development team about usability errors with their software. We also learn about design elements and features of the system that exhibited high levels of usability. Sometimes we learn that there was a question that arose during a usability test and which might need to be included with the next round of usability testing.

36. In which scenarios you should not perform usability testing? (d)

 (a) When the study cannot be accommodated within the lab space
 (b) When the study results will not be used to improve the system or make a purchasing decision
 (c) When typical participants cannot be recruited for the study
 (d) All of the above

 There are many circumstances when usability testing is not the best option. This includes when the study cannot be accommodated in the lab space. For example, if you were testing the process of taking a patient to the operating room. As we stated earlier, we should not undertake a study where the results will not be used or when we cannot find typical participants to be recruited to our study.

37. All of the following are linkages between patient safety and usability of clinical systems except? (c)

 (a) Confusing labels on the screen
 (b) Inability to link together relevant clinical data
 (c) Usability errors identified in a usability study
 (d) Unpleasant looking screens (Graphical User Interfaces)

 Usability errors that are identified during a usability study should be addressed and therefore would not lead to medical error. The other examples are situations that have predisposed patients to medical error. This includes confusing labels, and the position of data not allowing the identification of data that needs to be used concomitantly. A special case is unappealing interfaces, which can predispose the user to become distracted and therefore less aware of important information necessary for the appropriate provision of care.

38. The Human-Centred Design development lifecycle is? (b)

 (a) ISO 12207
 (b) ISO 13407
 (c) ISO 17117
 (d) ISO 9000

 The International Standards Organization standard ISO 13407 is the standard for the human-centred design development lifecycle. ISO 12207 is the software quality assurance lifecycle which deals with the recommendations for effective and efficient software development. ISO TS 17117 is the standard for quality indicators for healthcare terminologies. The ISO 9000 standards are a set of standards that are rapidly balloted and implemented for issues that require rapid standardization of quality management systems as they have important pressing use cases. These standards are process rather than device standards.

39. Usability of systems is composed of all except? (a)

    (a) Ease of error correction
    (b) Efficient to use
    (c) Subjectively pleasing
    (d) Few errors

    Usability of systems includes that they are efficient to use, have few errors and are subjectively pleasing. Usability would also include easy to learn and easy to remember. Ease of error correction is a functionality issue and is not a usability issue.

40. Types of human factors engineering include all except? (c)

    (a) Low fidelity prototyping
    (b) Contextual inquiry
    (c) Expert evaluation
    (d) Competitive usability evaluation

    Expert evaluations are sometimes important but does not constitute a usability evaluation, even if the expert is a well-regarded exert in the field or someone with a long history of experience. Low fidelity prototyping, contextual inquiry and competitive usability evaluations are all types of usability studies.

41. Usability engineering is? (b)

    (a) A usability laboratory
    (b) A process
    (c) A randomized controlled trial
    (d) An observational study

    Often after a laboratory is constructed outsiders and workers in the field alike often equate the lab itself with the process of usability testing. For example, we have a lab so doing usability study is not an uncommon sentiment. However, the most important component necessary to obtain valid usability study results we need to adhere to the usability methodology which is a process not a space. Both observational studies and randomized controlled trials (RCTs) can be accomplished within the usability setting.

Chapter 4
Knowledge Representation and the Logical Basis of Ontology

Peter L. Elkin and Steven H. Brown

Ontology as an outgrowth of the field of philosophy became a focus of application in healthcare terminologies in the 1990s and represents an important advance to the field. The increased rigor that formal definitions bring to terminologies improves our methodology in several distinct ways. First, it allows us to auto-classify the terminology which enables us to appropriately classify all concepts to all of the hierarchies to which they should belong. Second, it allows us to identify collisions or case where two concepts have the same formal definitions. This should lead to further definition of at least one of the concepts or combining the two concepts into one prior to release of that version of the terminology. Third, it allows us to reason

P. L. Elkin (✉)
Department of Biomedical Informatics, Jacobs School of Medicine and Biomedical Sciences, University at Buffalo, State University of New York, Buffalo, NY, USA

Internal Medicine, Jacobs School of Medicine and Biomedical Sciences, University at Buffalo, State University of New York, Buffalo, NY, USA

Surgery, Jacobs School of Medicine and Biomedical Sciences, University at Buffalo, State University of New York, Buffalo, NY, USA

Pathology and Anatomical Sciences, Jacobs School of Medicine and Biomedical Sciences, University at Buffalo, State University of New York, Buffalo, NY, USA

Psychiatry, Jacobs School of Medicine and Biomedical Sciences, University at Buffalo, State University of New York, Buffalo, NY, USA

Orthopedics, Jacobs School of Medicine and Biomedical Sciences, University at Buffalo, State University of New York, Buffalo, NY, USA
e-mail: elkinp@buffalo.edu;
http://medicine.buffalo.edu/departments/biomedical-informatics.html

S. H. Brown
Department of Veterans Affairs, Office of Health Informatics, Knowledge Based Systems, Washington, DC, USA

Department of Biomedical Informatics, Vanderbilt University, Nashville, TN, USA
e-mail: steven.brown@va.gov

P. L. Elkin (ed.), *Terminology, Ontology and their Implementations*, Health Informatics, https://doi.org/10.1007/978-3-031-11302-4_4

or operate on the content of the terminology. This includes asking questions of the terminology such as is a concept subsumed by another concept within the terminology or is a relationship between two concepts valid for that combination of operands and specifications. The formal definitions allow us to formulate rules at the highest level within the hierarchy where they should apply and then to take advantage of the explosions to capture all of the relevant individual cases. This mathematically represents the transitive reflexive closure on subsumption. As an example, it might include all forms of *Asthma* including the root concept, *Asthma* itself and its subtypes such as *Exercise-induced Asthma*.

To understand knowledge representation is to learn the basic principles of the field in addition to the logics that can be used to represent knowledge. This is independent of domain until one actually wishes to implement a knowledge representation system. In the case of terminologies, these often take the form of an instantiation of an ontology that relies heavily on domain expertise. By imbuing the terminology with the tenants and principles of the discipline, we create a knowledge-based system that can work with the users to help teach and improve knowledge in our case at the point of care.

The specific knowledge representation systems used as exemplars in this chapter are some of the more widely used and discussed systems available today. By learning their logics and purpose, we provide the reader with the background necessary to develop, select, and implement formal healthcare terminologies. As healthcare terminologies become large, it becomes more important that they are written and structured in accordance with knowledge representation principles and logics. As we learn more about healthcare and the implementation of informatics systems in the practice, we will evolve our logical underpinnings to be capable of asking ever more complex questions of our clinical data. As our clinical decision support systems advance, they will take greater advantage of this capability and help clinicians practice safer and more effective medicine.

Questions

1. A terminology is just another name for an ontology? False

   (a) True
   (b) False

   An ontology is a formally defined terminology. This requires that the ontology meet specific logical criteria that provides the foundation for meaning within the terminology and in its usage. The presence of computable definitions allows reasoners to operate on the terminology. After data has been instantiated in clinical records, the logical basis of ontology provides us with the means to reason over patient data and to cluster that data in a clinically relevant fashion.

2. An ontology is: (d)

   (a) A formal representation of the knowledge in a domain
   (b) The Web Ontology Language
   (c) A terminology with computable definitions
   (d) a and c
   (e) a, b, and c

Ontologies have formal definitions which are computable in a domain of knowledge. The Web Ontology Language (OWL) is a knowledge representation system that allows the instantiation of terminological and ontological information but is not itself an ontology. Therefore, the correct answer is (d).

3. The UMLS stands for? (c)

   (a) The Uniform Medical Logic System
   (b) The Uniform Medical Language System
   (c) The Unified Medical Language System
   (d) The Unified Medical Logic System

   The acronym UMLS was coined by the National Library of Medicine at the National Institutes of Health and stands for the Unified Medical Language System.

4. All of these are knowledge representation systems except: (b)

   (a) K-Rep
   (b) UMLS
   (c) OWL
   (d) KL-One

   The UMLS is a Metathesaurus and has a Knowledge Source Server but is not in itself a knowledge representation system. K-Rep or the Knowledge Representation system, the Web Ontology Language (OWL) and KL-One are all description logic-based knowledge representation systems.

5. Part of relations are defined in philosophy as a: (d)

   (a) Ontology
   (b) Topology
   (c) Metrology
   (d) Mereology

   Mereology is the study of part of relationships in a domain of expertise, in our case health care. Ontology is the study of meaning. Topology is the study of form or shapes. There are many topological principles of importance in Health Informatics but it does not specifically relate to part of relationships. Metrology is the science of measurement and comes from the Greek "metron."

6. Description logics are: (d)

   (a) Formal methods for defining concepts in an ontology
   (b) Provide a basis to auto-classify a formal terminology
   (c) Allow the specification of semantic triples
   (d) All of the above

   Description logics (DL) are formal methods for defining concepts in an ontology. They provide a basis for a DL reasoner to auto-classify the formal terminology. DLs specifically provide the ability to represent knowledge as sets of semantic triples. These triples can and often are used to connect concepts throughout the terminology where appropriate. They are also used to create description logic definitions for both pre-coordinated and post-coordinated concepts.

   Therefore, (d) all of the above is the correct answer.

7. All are true of description logics except? (b)

   (a) Subsets of first order predicate logics
   (b) Allow the specification of initial conditions
   (c) Allow the generation of directed acyclic graphs
   (d) All of the above

   Description logics (DLs) are all proper subsets of first order predicate logic. One can use description logics to create directed acyclic graphs (DAGs); however, not all DAGs can be reduced to a description logic representation. DLs do not allow the modeler to specify initial conditions whereas other formalisms such as conceptual graphs do include that capability which comes with some cost in terms of complexity.
8. Conceptual graphs are? (d)

   (a) Subsets of first order predicate logic
   (b) Allow the specification of initial conditions
   (c) Allow the generation of directed acyclic graphs
   (d) b and c
   (e) a, b, and c

   As conceptual graphs are capable of representing context as at least second order logic, they are not proper subsets of first order logic. They are capable of specifying initial conditions and of course allow the generation of DAGs, this capacity which is often why they would be selected as a formalism for terminological knowledge representation.
9. In modeling structural analysis has all these views except? (b)

   (a) Data view
   (b) Modeling view
   (c) Functional view
   (d) Dynamic view

   Structural analysis has three views; the data view that represents the physical representation of the data, the functional view which represents the purpose of the data, and the dynamic view that shows how the information can change and interact over time.
10. In the Unified Modeling Language protected classes are? (a)

   (a) Only accessible by the class members and members of any subclass
   (b) Only accessible by the class members alone
   (c) Protected from access by other members of the class
   (d) Protected from access by members of their subclasses

   Like most object-oriented programming languages the Unified Modeling Language (UML) has the provision to specify protected classes of information. In UML, this serves to wall off information that can be used differently in different contexts. Therefore, in this model a specific concept will have this specified meaning. This meaning would be shared by the protected class itself and any subclasses that are generated would also have the ability to access and use that shared meaning. However, classes that are not subclasses of the protected class would not have access to that meaning and would not be constrained to that meaning. For example, in a pediatric population the concept "Chest Pain" might have different inferencing applied to it and therefore require different methods than in an adult population.

11. Foreign keys? (c)

    (a) Map information from one language to another
    (b) Open security access to tables
    (c) Connect two tables within a database by a common data column
    (d) Open security access between databases

    A foreign key is a column in one database table that holds the match to the key in another table within the same database. Specifying columns as foreign keys creates constraints that require that the column entries exist as a key in the foreign table being referenced. These constraints help to normalize the database tables to protect against key references that do not exist (e.g., often this leads to the existence of data that is not fully defined). The foreign key references do not map information between languages, and they do not open security either to tables or databases.

12. The Object Control Language: (e)

    (a) Allows designers to place constraints on operations
    (b) Allows designers to assign invariants to objects
    (c) Allows designers to assign pre- and postconditions to methods
    (d) a and b
    (e) a, b, and c

    The Object Control Language (OCL) is a standard developed by the Object Management Group as a method to write constraints for UML models. OCL allows designers to place constraints on operations and to assign preconditions and postconditions to methods this specifies how actors in the model can and cannot be used. Therefore, (e) is the correct answer.

13. Invariants in OCL are? (b)

    (a) Things that are always true about classes but not their subclasses (the transitive closure of subsumption)
    (b) Things that are always true about classes and their subclasses (the transitive reflexive closure of subsumption)
    (c) Things that are not true for their class but are true for their subclasses
    (d) Things that are not true about classes or their subclasses

    An invariant is a condition that is always true for a class or any of its subclasses. The transitive component of the transitive reflexive closure of subsumption is that all the children or subtypes of the class are included in the constraint (meaning that the constraint applies to all the subclasses of a class). The reflexive closure of subsumption means that the constraint also applies to the reference class (e.g., *Asthma* as a class of disorders is itself included in the class of types of *Asthma*). Therefore, (b) is the correct answer.

14. Which statement is true regarding OCL? **(c)**

    (a) A package is a type of model
    (b) A model is made up of multiple packages
    (c) A model is a type of package
    (d) A package cannot contain a model

    Packages in OCL contain one or more models that are to be referenced together. Although models can serve as packages, they can be a container for models and not be a model themselves. Therefore, (a) is not always true and therefore (c) is true that a model is a type of package.

15. Which statement(s) are true regarding OWL? (d)

    (a) It is a description logic-based knowledge representation language
    (b) It is the language of the semantic Web
    (c) It is limited to the representation of first order predicate logic
    (d) All of the above
    (e) None of the above

    The Web Ontology Language (OWL) is a description logic-based knowledge representation language optimized for use on the World Wide Web. In point of fact, it is the language of the semantic Web standardized and popularized by the w3c who developed the http protocol and the format for html pages that are used widely today. It can be written using the RDFS XML format, and it is a proper subset of first order predicate logic. Therefore, (d), all of the above, is the correct answer.

16. All of the following are species of the OWL language except? (b)

    (a) OWL Full
    (b) OWL Bright
    (c) OWL Description Logic
    (d) OWL Lite

    OWL represents the language instead of WOL which would be the acronym as it is fun to make reference to the bird that bears the same name. At one time, there was talk of creating types such as Barn OWLs, Screech Owls, etc. The language took a more pragmatic turn when it specified OWL Full and then created OWL DL as a proper subset of OWL Full and limited OWL to a more decidable subset of the more expressive language. OWL Lite was developed to service the need of developers that wanted to move ontologies into a Web-based environment but had minimal needs for inferencing. This lightweight version of OWL is a proper subset of OWL DL and contains machinery for formal definitions, but the constraint mechanisms and operations are limited in comparison to OWL DL and OWL Full.

17. OWL stands for? (d)

    (a) The Ontology Web Language
    (b) The Open Web Language
    (c) The Web Ontology Learning System
    (d) The Web Ontology Language

    OWL stands for the Web Ontology Language and not the Ontology Web Language which would be accurate but not as much fun. Therefore, (d) is the correct answer.

18. The difference between OWL Full and OWL DL is? (b)

    (a) OWL DL does not have the full set of operations
    (b) OWL DL does not allow same name for objects and properties
    (c) OWL DL has a description logic underpinning the language
    (d) OWL DL is missing the ability to specify invariants

    OWL DL differs from OWL Full in that it does not allow designers to use the same name for an object as an object property or a datatype or a datatype property. The names in these four classes of objects are mutually exclusive in OWL DL where they are not in OWL Full. Allowing this to be designed permits some higher order logical expressions and reasoning but can lead to some questions not being decidable in our lifetimes as the complexity can go up exponentially by using this capability of OWL Full. OWL DL has the full set of operations of OWL Full and is by definition a description logic formalism. You can specify invariants with the OWL DL language. Therefore, (b) is the correct answer.

19. OWL can be represented as all of the following except? (d)

    (a) RDF triples
    (b) Abstract Syntax
    (c) XML
    (d) Conceptual graph with pre-conditions

    The Web Ontology Language (OWL) can be represented in its Abstract Syntax, or as RDF triples which is an XML formalism also standardized by the w3c. Conceptual graphs are a logical formalism which is competitive with description logics such as OWL. With conceptual graphs a logical construction has the ability to specify initial conditions also called pre-conditions.

20. The following is/are true about ontologies? (e)

    (a) A level one ontology is domain independent
    (b) A level two ontology is domain dependent
    (c) A level three ontology inherits the constraints of the level two and level one ontologies
    (d) A level three ontology is composed of both classes and instances
    (e) All of the above

    There are three levels of ontologies. The level one is domain independent. These are things that are true about the whole world, by definition. Level two ontologies are things that are true about a specific domain. The level two ontologies must be consistent with the level one ontology. Level three ontologies are methods for representing detailed information about the domain which can be instantiated in, for example, a patient's clinical record. This corresponds to the leaf nodes and some of the categorical or organizing nodes within a clinical terminology. The level three ontology includes atomic concepts, pre-coordinated concepts and post-coordinated concepts. Where to draw the line between the level two and level three ontology can be based on the judgment of the ontology designer. However, the level three ontology must be consistent and constrained by both the level two and level one ontologies to which it relates. Because the terminological concepts can be stored in patient records, the instance data is also part of the ontology and later can feed back to the ontology with information such as frequency data that can be important to the usability of the terminology as an interface terminology. Therefore, the correct answer is (e) all of the above are true.

Chapter 5
Compositionality

Peter L. Elkin and Steven H. Brown

This chapter concerns itself with the method and rules for constructing post-coordinated or compositional expressions using clinical terminologies. It is clear that only certain types of concepts can be the operand or the specification in the semantic triple. This is important to ensure that we only generate valid semantic relationships. This would correspond to the referent and the proposition. For example:

Streptococcal pneumoniae	HasEtiology	*Streptococcus pneumoniae*
Operand	Relation	Specification
Infectious disorder	HasEtiology	Organism

P. L. Elkin (✉)
Department of Biomedical Informatics, Jacobs School of Medicine and Biomedical Sciences, University at Buffalo, State University of New York, Buffalo, NY, USA

Internal Medicine, Jacobs School of Medicine and Biomedical Sciences, University at Buffalo, State University of New York, Buffalo, NY, USA

Surgery, Jacobs School of Medicine and Biomedical Sciences, University at Buffalo, State University of New York, Buffalo, NY, USA

Pathology and Anatomical Sciences, Jacobs School of Medicine and Biomedical Sciences, University at Buffalo, State University of New York, Buffalo, NY, USA

Psychiatry, Jacobs School of Medicine and Biomedical Sciences, University at Buffalo, State University of New York, Buffalo, NY, USA

Orthopedics, Jacobs School of Medicine and Biomedical Sciences, University at Buffalo, State University of New York, Buffalo, NY, USA
e-mail: elkinp@buffalo.edu;
http://medicine.buffalo.edu/departments/biomedical-informatics.html

S. H. Brown
Department of Veterans Affairs, Office of Health Informatics, Knowledge Based Systems, Washington, DC, USA

Department of Biomedical Informatics, Vanderbilt University, Nashville, TN, USA
e-mail: steven.brown@va.gov

P. L. Elkin (ed.), *Terminology, Ontology and their Implementations*, Health Informatics, https://doi.org/10.1007/978-3-031-11302-4_5

These sorts of rules can be augmented with decisions about which concepts are Kernel concepts (the main point or central concept in the compositional expression), Modifiers, Qualifiers, Severity, or Laterality. Rules can be created for the automated construction of expressions with high reliability. The principles necessary for this type of construction are provided in this chapter.

Questions

1. What is compositionality? (b)

   (a) The ability to compose single concepts within a terminology
   (b) Compositions are expressions made up of more than one concept where all pairs are joined by relationships
   (c) Compositions are expressions not found in the original terminology
   (d) Compositions are pre-coordinated concepts

   Compositional expressions often are expressed within a logical formalism such as a description logic language. These expressions bind two or more concepts together where each concept pair is joined together through a relationship or semantic link. These expressions can be either pre-coordinated or post-coordinated expressions. The ability to compose single concepts and to create pre-coordinated expressions or as in (c) post-coordinated expressions are just part of the functions provided by compositional expressions. Therefore, (b) is the correct answer.

2. Acceptable formalisms for defining compositional expressions are? (e)

   (a) OWL
   (b) Conceptual graphs
   (c) Description logics
   (d) DAGs
   (e) All of the above

   Description logics and conceptual graphs are both logical formalisms capable of expressing compositional structures and semantics. OWL is a description logic formalism and Directed Acyclic Graphs (DAGs) can be constructed from either conceptual graphs or a description logic representation. Therefore, the correct answer is (e) all of the above.

3. How many concepts does it take to represent billions of clinical utterances using a compositional terminology? (a)

   (a) $<10^6$
   (b) $<10^{10}$
   (c) $<10^9$
   (d) $<10^8$
   (e) $<10^7$

   The power of composition is the expressivity that comes with the ability to combine concepts to create more specific expressions. These expressions can be arbitrarily long and can contain a large number of concepts. In our experience, we have seen actual compositional expressions with as many as 13 concepts representing complex clinical notions. Once constructed these expressions can be reused and referred to as if they were one concept. By growing the terminology by actual constructions derived from clinical practice, we limit the number of constructions from a cross product of the various semantics over the practical number of concepts in a construction (a very large number) to the notions that are actually referred to with some frequency with the use of the compositional terminology. These compositional expressions can be submitted to the terminology developers for inclusion in future releases of the terminology for the convenience of other users of that terminology. SNOMED CT has ~291,000 active concepts in its July 2010 release and can be used to represent billions of notions. Based on these principles and our data from SNOMED CT, it would take less than a million concepts in a compositional terminology to represent literally billions of clinical utterances. Therefore, (a) is the correct answer.

4. How many concepts does it take to represent billions of clinical utterances using a non-compositional terminology? (c)

   (a) $<10^6$
   (b) $<10^{10}$
   (c) $<10^9$
   (d) $<10^8$
   (e) $<10^7$

   In a non-compositional terminology, the expressivity scales with the number of concepts in the terminology. Given that we do not know how many clinical utterances are expressing the same ideas the only safe answer is (c) less than a billion concepts.

5. The operand in a compositional expression is? (c)

   (a) The operator
   (b) The relationship
   (c) The main concept of the expression
   (d) The refining characteristic

   The main concept is a compositional expression becomes the operand. This has also been called by some in the computational linguistics field as the "head" concept. By building parse trees from concepts rather than words, we have the advantage of the formal definitions to anchor the meaning of the expression as decisions are made regarding its construction.

6. The specification of the compositional expression is? (d)

   (a) The operator
   (b) The relationship
   (c) The main concept of the expression
   (d) The refining characteristic

   Specifications in compositional expressions refine the meaning of the operand. Operators and relationships are used to link concepts to one another. The operand is the main concept in the expression. Therefore, (d) is the correct answer.

7. Having independent semantics means? (b)

    (a) That only one semantic can be used in a compositional expression
    (b) That the semantics used are non-overlapping in meaning
    (c) That the concepts are non-overlapping in meaning with the semantics
    (d) That the semantics are defined by terms in the terminology

    Semantic independence is the notion that all of the semantics used in your terminology are non-overlapping in meaning. This means that no reasonable expert could construct a concept with the same meaning using two different semantics. This is difficult as a designer of the terminology has to have the forethought to recognize every possible way that the semantic relations can be used to create compositions that have the same meaning. The best way to avoid this source of ambiguity is to limit your relationships to those that are well defined and narrowly focused and as much as possible their meaning should be orthogonal to each other. As an example, the original semantics from SNOMED CT were orthogonal (HasMorphology, HasFindingSite, and HasEtiology). Therefore, (b) is the correct answer. Answers (a) and (d) are simply not true. Answer (c) refers to concepts rather than relations.
8. Uniformity of relations means? (d)

    (a) That the representational form of the relations is consistent
    (b) That uniformity is used in assigning names to relations
    (c) That relations are linked to concepts
    (d) That relations are applied everywhere they are applicable within the terminology

    Relations should be applied uniformly. This means that each relation is applied to every relevant definition in the terminology. So for example if infectious disorders should all have organisms, every infectious disease is defined by the relationship HasOrganism with the relevant organism or class of organisms specified. The logical expression would also hold the existential or universal quantifier appropriate to the specification. So if it was any bacterial infection, for example, the existential quantifier "some" would be appropriate and if it was "*Streptococcus pneumoniae*" it would be the universal quantifier as all *S. pneumoniae* are included rather than just one of a set of bacterial infections. Therefore, (d) is the correct answer. The form of the names and the fact that the relations are linked to concepts does not fully define uniformity of relations.
9. Logical consistency means? (c)

    (a) That you use the same logic throughout the development of the terminology
    (b) That you use the same logic for the use of post-coordinated compositional expressions
    (c) That you use the same logic for the development and use of the terminology
    (d) That you use the same logic as a DL classifier and a conceptual graph classifier

In terminological systems, it is very important to keep in mind that the meaning of information is only retained if it is logically equivalent between its source and destination or between two individual reviewers. Logical consistency requires that the same methods of logical construction be used to identify and store the data as to access the data once stored. It is also true that this requires that the methods used to create the pre-coordinated concepts within the terminology are the exact same methods used to create post-coordinated expressions. Therefore, answer (c) is the correct answer. Answers (a) and (b) are incomplete and answer (d) is a method for constructing the logic but not the logical system of the terminology itself.

10. Semantic normalization is present when you are able to? (a)

    (a) Identify all of the pre-coordinated and post-coordinated concepts with the same meaning
    (b) Identify all the pre-coordinated concepts with the same meaning as an atomic concept
    (c) Identify all the atomic concepts with the same meaning as a pre-coordinated concept
    (d) Identify all the atomic concepts with the same meaning as a post-coordinated concept

    Semantic normalization is an important and central notion in the field of ontology and healthcare terminology. Semantic normalization requires that you can tell everywhere in the terminology including post-coordinations that have the same meaning. For example, if there are 15 ways to say "Appendicitis" in SNOMED CT, the system should be able to automatically detect that all 15 ways represent the same concept. This requires that one is able to identify all of the pre-coordinated and post-coordinated concepts with the same meaning. Therefore, (a) is the correct answer. Atomic concepts cannot by definition have the same meaning as either pre-coordinated or post-coordinated concepts. Therefore, answers (b), (c), and (d) are incorrect.

11. Computational normalization is when the classifier used to build the terminology is capable of auditing the terminology and its post-coordinated expressions? (a)

    (a) True
    (b) False
    (c) Unknown
    (d) Unknowable

    Computational normalization requires that the classifier is capable of auditing the meaning and auto-classifying the terminology including any post-coordinated expressions. Therefore, our statement (a) is true.

12. Colloquial normalization is when? (c)

    (a) Things that are commonly said are normalized
    (b) Normalization is used when it is practical to do so

   (c) Allowable grammar is limited to what can be normalized by the classifier
   (d) Normalization is limited to semantics that have worked in the past

   Colloquial normalization means that the allowable grammar is limited to what can be normalized by the classifier. This also means that the ability to use post-coordinated expressions rather than atomic or pre-coordinated concepts is limited by the capability of the classifier to normalize those constructions. This helps to prevent unrecognized ambiguity.

13. It is worthwhile creating a pre-coordinated concept in a terminology when? (d)

   (a) Experts think you should
   (b) The terminology looks more clinical with the concept
   (c) The terminology looks incomplete without the concept
   (d) You need to associate the concepts with other information in the terminology

   There are many good reasons for creating pre-coordinations in a terminology, even a reference terminology. A terminological reason for creating a pre-coordination is that you need to use that pre-coordinated concept in the definition of another concept. For example, *Colon Cancer* is a pre-coordination as it can be represented as *Malignant Neoplasm* HasFindingSite *Colon*. You may want to partially define *Iron Deficiency Anemia* as HasEtiology *Colon Cancer*. It is also useful for terminologies to appear sensible, such that an expert in the field can see the concepts that they expect in any given region of the hierarchy; however, this can also be accomplished through post-coordination and meaning takes precedence over form. Be careful not to create ambiguous expressions by staying within the logical boundaries of the representational formalism. Answer (d) is the best answer.

14. Creating a pre-coordinated compositional expression? (c)

   (a) Adds new knowledge to the terminology
   (b) Adds more information to the terminology
   (c) Does not add new knowledge to the terminology
   (d) Adds semantics to the terminology

   Pre-coordinations are made up of concepts and relationships from the terminology applied using a permissible logical formalism followed by the terminological design. Therefore, all possible pre-coordinations are capable of being represented as post-coordinations; therefore, pre-coordinated expressions do not add new or addition knowledge or semantics to the terminology. Therefore, answer (c) is correct.

15. When do you want to post-coordinate concepts? (d)

   (a) When the specification would apply to a large number of concepts
   (b) When the expression uses semantics which have high reliability of assignment
   (c) When forming an expression for "History of CABG"
   (d) All of the above

There are many important reasons for using post-coordination rather than pre-coordination in terminological development. One of the easiest ways to understand is that combining *Status-Post* with concepts such as *Acute Myocardial Infarction* is a useful post-coordination. Almost anything you have could have had in the past and therefore could be "*Status-Post*." This would close to double the size of the disorder's hierarchy and make maintenance of the terminology more difficult. Classification of the categories of the allowable operands and specifications for that relationship should be highly reliable. The expression "History of CABG" makes the same point as *S/P AMI* referenced above.

16. When using more than one terminology to form compositional expressions? (b)

    (a) It is important to delete all overlapping content from the larger terminology
    (b) It is important to normalize the content and semantics of each terminology
    (c) It is important to delete all the overlapping semantics from the larger terminology
    (d) It is important to delete the overlapping content from the smaller terminology

    In compositional systems, it should be possible to normalize the content and semantics of terminology. Special problems arise when expressions can be formed using concepts from multiple terminologies. This means that both the content and semantics need to be mapped including the formal definitions from each terminology. For example, if I want to use RxNorm to represent medications and SNOMED CT to represent clinical problems, I have an issue when I get to the concept *Penicillin Allergy* which is defined as HasMorphology *Hypersensitivity Reaction* and HasMedication *Penicillin* substance as a concept in SNOMED CT. Therefore, the normalization could only happen if the definition of penicillin allergy from the disorders hierarchy were mapped to RxNorm in addition to the medications being mapped to one another. Deleting the overlapping content and/or semantics from one terminology will cause problems as that terminology will now not properly auto-classify. Therefore, (b) is the correct answer.

17. When using multiple terminologies in compositional expressions? (c)

    (a) It is important to examine the concepts from both terminologies
    (b) It is important to map together the concepts from each terminology together
    (c) It is important to map together the concepts and their description logic references
    (d) It is important not to be fooled by the name description logic

    Compositional expressions have to retain their meaning and be consistent with the meaning of the concepts from their source vocabularies. This requires that you map together both the concepts and their formal definitions (e.g., description logic references). Therefore, (c) is the correct answer. Answers (a) and (b) are only partially correct and answer (d) is not relevant.

18. Composition improves SNOMED CT's coverage of clinical problems by? (c)

    (a) 21%
    (b) 31%
    (c) 41%
    (d) 51%

    In one study noted in this chapter, the addition of post-coordination to SNOMED CT improved the content coverage for clinical problems from 51.4% to 92.3%. Therefore, the closest answer is (c).
19. Compositionality increases terminological expressivity by? (b)

    (a) 10^5
    (b) 10^4
    (c) 10^3
    (d) 10^2

    As we found that SNOMED CT can represent billions of clinical utterances with only ~291,000 concepts, the addition of composition improves SNOMED CT's expressivity by 10^4. Therefore, (b) is the correct answer.
20. A safe compositional expression is one that? (a)

    (a) Is logically well formed and is capable of being normalized
    (b) Has already been normalized with the terminology
    (c) Has been written using a description logic representation
    (d) Has no collisions with pre-coordinated concepts from the terminology

    Safety in the creation of compositional expressions relates to the danger of creating unrecognized ambiguous or redundant expressions. This can be prevented if the logical formalism and content of each construction is well formed and consistent with best practice. This will lead to the ability to normalize the terminology and will protect against unrecognized ambiguity and redundancy. This is what we call a "safe" compositional expression. Therefore, (a) is the correct answer. The process of normalization without being confident that all the content and semantics are accounted for in the normalization process will not be guaranteed to lead to the safe generation of compositional expressions. The use of a description logic does not guarantee that this level of normalization is possible. The post-coordinations should not have collisions with either atomic or pre-coordinated concepts. Atomic concepts can collide with post-coordinations when they are not truly atomic however the designers have not fully defined the concept. This can occur when relations and propositions are not applied everywhere in the terminology where they should be applied based on their relevance to that concept.

Chapter 6
The Place of Referent Tracking in Biomedical Informatics

Werner Ceusters

Questions

1. An electronic medical record (EMR) contains structured data in the form of codes that are picked from a coding system which uses an unambiguous and standardized terminology. True or false: are therefore these data unambiguous? False

   Terminologies and coding systems allow users thereof to understand what the terms and codes mean. When, for example, the SNOMED CT code "254588001|Polyp of intestine (disorder)|" is used in a patient's EMR to express a diagnosis, and if this diagnosis is correct, then this code may be taken to mean that there is in the body of that patient some entity for which the code and the corresponding term provide an appropriate description. But what is missing is which entity the code is precisely about. If there is only one such polyp, the code is about that one, but if there is more than one, it cannot be determined about which one the statement was made, unless the statement would include a unique identifier not just for the term, but for the entity in the patient's body to which the code applies. Data are not only ambiguous when they are expressed by means of ill-defined codes or use of homonymous terms, but also when they not uniquely identify the precise entities to which the codes are ascribed.
2. What is meant by "referent ambiguity"? (b)

   (a) The meaning of a predicate used to describe an entity is not clear
   (b) Which entity the predicate is about is not clear

W. Ceusters (✉)
Department of Biomedical Informatics, Jacobs School of Medicine and Biomedical Sciences, University at Buffalo, Buffalo, NY, USA

Department of Psychiatry, Jacobs School of Medicine and Biomedical Sciences, University at Buffalo, Buffalo, NY, USA

P. L. Elkin (ed.), *Terminology, Ontology and their Implementations*, Health Informatics, https://doi.org/10.1007/978-3-031-11302-4_6

Biomedical terminologies take care of what can be predicated in a standardized and relatively unambiguous way, at least in a sense that the terms they contain give a good idea of what happened somewhere on the side of the patient. But they come not equipped with a mechanism to specify the concrete referent of a predicate. Specifying what an entity is about is the responsibility of the author of a predicate. Failing to specify to which entity one refers may lead to referent ambiguity.

3. Which of the following SNOMED CT codes is least prone to referent ambiguity? (c)

   (a) 273367002|Clinical dementia rating scale (assessment scale)|
   (b) 716546001|Moss Attention Rating Scale score (observable entity)|
   (c) 273538004|IOWA low back rating scale (assessment scale)|
   (d) 718737000|Assessment using Zung self-rating depression scale (procedure)|

   Least prone to referent ambiguity is "IOWA low back rating scale (assessment scale)" as the term designates a precise rating scale. Referent ambiguity might arise if several versions would have been developed, while still the same name would be used for the scale. The other three codes require explicit referencing when used. "Clinical dementia rating scale (assessment scale)" may refer to any scale which rates dementia. "Moss Attention Rating Scale score (observable entity)" does not refer to the Moss Attention Rating Scale, but a score obtained on that scale; it requires referencing which score precisely (the one obtained by patient John or by patient Suzy?). Of similar nature is "Assessment using Zung self-rating depression scale (procedure)": it should refer to the precise procedure in which the Zung scale was used, for example, on patient X at that date and time.

4. A data analyst extracts from all patients described in some EMR system the diagnoses that have been entered together with the dates at which these diagnoses were entered. For some patient X, he obtains the following list:

   02/03/1985: 92065004|Benign neoplasm of colon (disorder)|
   04/23/1986: 92065004|Benign neoplasm of colon (disorder)|
   03/18/1987: 363406005|Malignant neoplasm of colon (disorder)|

   How many colon neoplasms are these diagnoses descriptions of assuming the diagnoses were all correct at the time that they were made? (a)

   (a) At least one
   (b) At least two
   (c) At least three

   In 1985, there must have been at least one neoplasm as others might have been missed. For the diagnosis made in 1986, one has to guess whether it is a confirmation of the first diagnosis, or whether it is about a second neoplasm in the colon which either was already there in 1985, but missed, or came into existence after the first diagnosis was made. In 1987, it might be that an existing and previously as benign described neoplasm was found to have become malignant, or it might be one that developed after the second diagnosis. It is because of referent ambiguity, and the assumption about the correctness of all diagnoses, that the correct answer is "at least one." How many exactly is impossible to tell.

5. Knowledge representation system X is designed to satisfy the following requirements. Which one violates the principles of Referent Tracking? (b)

   (a) An author may only enter a predicate in X when he has sufficient arguments to believe that the predicate is true
   (b) X must be capable of accepting predicates about anything perceivable or conceivable
   (c) X may contain predicates contradicting each other
   (d) X must keep track of the provenance of predicates

   The phrase "anything perceivable or conceivable" comes from a series of ISO terminology standards (e.g., https://www.iso.org/obp/ui/#iso:std:iso:1087:ed-2:v1:en) and functions therein as the definition for "object." Referent Tracking does not allow predicates to be "about" what is merely conceived and does or did not exist. Such predicates are about nothing at all. Of course, the conception itself, i.e., a belief, a type of cognitive representation, is real and predicates can be made about it: there cannot be a predicate "about" flogiston in an RTS, but there can be predicates about people who believed that flogiston existed.

6. Referent Tracking and the Basic Formal Ontology are designed on the basis of the same ontological principles. Which of the following assertions is nevertheless false? (c)

   (a) Representations in BFO and in RT are faithful to reality
   (b) The structure of representations in BFO and in RT mimic the structure of reality
   (c) Representations in BFO and in RT are about universals, collections of particulars and individual particulars

   BFO uses the names of universals to represent what is true for all particulars that are instances of some universal. BFO does not assert anything about specific particulars. Typical RT representations in contrast are about specific particulars.

7. Order the following representations to the extent they mimic the structure of reality of what they are representations of, i.e., a molecule of what is commonly known as *drinking alcohol*. Order from lowest to highest degree of mimicking (e, c, b, a, d or e, c, a, b, d)

   (a) Ethanol molecule
   (b) C_2H_5OH
   (c) Ethyl alcohol molecule
   (d) CH_3–CH_2–OH
   (e) C_2H_6O

Of this list, the representation which mimics the structure of reality most closely is CH_3–CH_2–OH. This is because it represents explicitly the type and quantities of the individual atoms of which an ethanol molecule is composed, as well as implicitly (one has to understand the syntactical conventions for combining chemical formulae in this notation) how the atoms are bound. Next comes “ethanol molecule” but it requires to understand how the word “ethanol” is formed, i.e., as a composition defined by IUPAC for a compound consisting of an alkyl group with two carbon atoms (prefix “eth-”), having a single bond between them (infix “-an-”) and an attached functional group –OH group. This is also reflected in the formula C_2H_5OH which therefor can be considered to be mimicking to the same degree. A bit less explicit is ‘ethyl alcohol”: “ethyl” represents the same molecule part as “eth – an” but “alcohol” is less informative than mentioning the extra “OH” group. Least mimicking of all is C_2H_6O as it provides no explicit structural information.

8. What are the four ontological distinctions that are essential to apply Referent Tracking correctly?

   (a) The distinction between representations, i.e., predicates and their components in particular, and what they are about, i.e., their referents
   (b) The distinction between portions of reality which are specific (non-repeatable) and portions of reality which are generic (repeatable)
   (c) The distinction between continuants and occurrents
   (d) The distinction between dependent and independent entities

9. In the FHIR documentation, the following assertions about conditions can be found: (1) on the one hand that a condition is a *a clinical condition, problem, diagnosis, or other event, situation, issue, or clinical concept that has risen to a level of concern* and on the other hand that *conditions are frequently a result of a clinician’s assessment*. Which ontological distinction does FHIR here fail to make? (a)

   (a) The distinction between representations, i.e., predicates and their components in particular, and what they are about, i.e., their referents
   (b) The distinction between portions of reality which are specific (non-repeatable) and portions of reality which are generic (repeatable)
   (c) The distinction between continuants and occurrents
   (d) The distinction between dependent and independent entities

   The distinction between representations which result from a clinician’s assessment, and the referents of these representations, i.e., what the clinician would actually be assessing.

10. Under what condition is an identifier singularly unique? (a)

   (a) When the portion of reality it denotes is not denoted by another identifier
   (b) When the identifier denotes precisely one portion of reality

   Referent tracking aims numerically unique portions of reality to be referenced by identifiers that are *singularly* and *globally* unique within a single referent tracking system or a network of referent tracking systems that exchange information. An identifier is globally unique when it denotes precisely one portion of reality. An identifier is singularly unique when the portion of reality it denotes is not denoted by another identifier.

11. An RUI is a representation that denotes, i.e., identifies—or is intended to do so—a portion of reality in a *globally unique* way within the confines of an RTS. For most portions of reality, RUIs should ideally also be *singularly unique*. This can for some entities, although they are numerically unique, not always be guaranteed at the time the identifier is to be assigned. For what type of entities referenced in relational expressions, i.e., RT-tuples, is that almost always the case? (b)

    (a) Material entities
    (b) Temporal regions
    (c) Sites
    (d) Processes

    This happens often with identifiers for temporal regions because it is in most cases very hard, if not impossible, to determine whether two numerically distinct entities are related to two other numerically distinct entities within exactly the same temporal region.

12. Why is the extended EAV-tuple "(Jane Smith, hasLength, 6 feet, on 10/03/2009)" not compatible with Referent Tracking? (c)

    (a) "Feet" is not an ISO unit of measurement
    (b) The time specification is not precise enough as only a date is provided
    (c) Jane Smith's length is not uniquely identified

    Referent Tracking does not allow—modulo some precisely defined exceptions—the use of "shortcut" relations that relate, for example, a particular p to a universal U of which p is not an instance thereby bypassing reference to an existing particular q that is instance of U. The bypassed particular q here is Jane Smith's length, a quality which inheres in Jane Smith since her coming into existence, while changing from time to time in the sense that it becomes instance of another length universal. To be compatible with RT, the extended EAV-tuple should be replaced by two distinct ones, for example:
    (Jane Smith's length, inheresIn, Jane Smith, since 03/01/1980)
    (Jane Smith's length, instanceOf, length of 6 feet, on 10/03/2009)

13. Which tuple type from the following list is used to keep track of assertions in a Referent Tracking System? (b)

    (a) A-tuples
    (b) D-tuples
    (c) F-tuples
    (d) NtoN-tuples

    It is through A-tuples that identifiers are assigned to entities. NtoN-tuples describe relations between non-repeatable entities. F-tuples are used to assert the confidence an author has in the faithfulness of another tuple in the RTS. D-tuples are used to assert the addition or replacement of tuples of other types and are thus the ones that keep track of the assertions.

14. John was in 2020 correctly diagnosed with a benign brain tumor which accounted for the repeated headaches he suffered from for years. In 2021, the tumor was successfully removed and since then, he never had headache anymore. When this information would be registered in a Referent Tracking System, the presence of the tumor in John's head in 2020 and the absence of that tumor in John's head after his surgery, can each be expressed by means of an NtoN-tuple. Can such NtoN-tuple also be used to express that John has no headache anymore, yes or no? No

    (a) Yes
    (b) No

    No! Since John does not have a headache anymore, there is no headache to assign an identifier to while that is required for an NtoN-tuple. The correct tuple to use is an NtoR(−)-tuple that refers to a repeatable portion of reality rather than a non-repeatable one and that expresses that of all the instances of headache, there is none which inheres in John. With an NtoN-tuple, it would be only possible to express that John does not have a prior headache—thus an identified one—anymore. That does not exclude that he has other instances of headache.

15. Which quality construct out of the following list can be applied to a specific type of representation that the others in the list cannot? (d)

    (a) Signal-to-noise
    (b) Fragmentation
    (c) Concordance
    (d) Correctness
    (e) Completeness

    Correctness is the only quality construct out of the list that can be applied to individual predicates. All the others require a collection of predicates.

16. Is it possible for a collection of tuples not to be adequately faithful to reality despite all of its individual tuples being adequately faithful to reality? Yes

    (a) Yes
    (b) No

    It is possible. A representation is *adequately faithful* to reality whenever it is faithful to reality at a level of granularity that is equal or more precise than what is required for the purposes for which the representation is used. When a representation consists of a collection of tuples, it might very well be that each tuple is adequately faithful to reality, but that the collection is not, for instance when the collection is incomplete, has high signal-to-noise, or contains tuples which are not adequately faithful *throughout* reality.

17. The SNOMED CT concept "|Removal of nail (procedure)|" is formally fully defined as:
    === |Removal (procedure)| +
        |Procedure on nail (procedure)| :
            {|Procedure site - Direct (attribute)| = |Nail unit structure (body structure)|,
            |Method (attribute)| = |Removal - action (qualifier value)| }

    If this concept were selected by a clinician to register in the EMR of a patient that this procedure was applied, and the EMR uses RT tuples to encode patient data based on a BFO perspective on the SNOMED CT concept-based ontology, what is the minimum number of new globally and singularly unique RUIs that would have to be assigned? (c)

    (a) 0
    (b) 1
    (c) 2
    (d) 3
    (e) 4

    Because the patient would have already been assigned an RUI, two additional ones would be created: one for the procedure and one for the nail. Although the SNOMED CT definition refers to two procedure types, i.e., "procedure on nail" and "removal," there is only one procedure instance involved: that what is done is both an instance of removal and an instance of (the defined class) "procedure on nail."
18. Out of the following list of BFO 2.0 types, what must be the type of non-repeatable entity #12 for tuple *NtoN-321< '-', r-45, {#12,#56}, '-', '-'>* to be of a correct form? (d)

    (a) Independent continuant
    (b) Site
    (c) Role
    (d) Process

    NtoN tuples are used to describe whether a specific relationship obtains between two non-repeatable entities. Tuple NtoN-321 does not specify a temporal region, so both relata can only be occurrents. The only occurrent type in the list is "process." Although this was the case for BFO 2.0, BFO2020 does include relations between continuants that are not time-indexed.
19. A Referent Tracking Database (RTDB) serving as back-end for an EMR contains the following RT-tuple: *NtoR#-2301< '+', inst, #-786, OGMS:acute disease course, '-', '-'>*. During a follow-up visit of the patient about whom the tuple is registered, additional data is entered which by the RTS is translated into the following tuple and then assessed for faithfulness to reality: *NtoR#-2941< '+', inst, #-786, OGMS:chronic disease course, '-', '-'>*. What should a properly designed RTS do? (b)

(a) Add a D-tuple to the RTDB reflecting when and by whom tuple NtoR#-2941 was added
(b) Alert the clinician that NtoR#-2941 is incompatible with NtoR#-2301 and suggest plausible alternatives

NtoR tuples are used to assert the type of an entity. Tuple NtoR#-2301 claims entity #-786 to be of the type OGMS:acute disease course, thus a process as can also be inferred from the absence of time-indexing in the tuple. Tuple NtoR#-2941 claims the very same entity to be of a different type, i.e., chronic disease course. That is however impossible as processes cannot change type. The proper action for the RTS is to ask the clinician for a resolution and suggest possible alternatives.

20. What is the purpose of the NtoC-tuple? (c)

(a) To make assertions of which the faithfulness to reality is uncertain
(b) To declare an entity to instantiate a type present in an upper ontology
(c) To classify entities following the provisions of a coding and classification system

Confidence in the faithfulness of a tuple T can be expressed by referencing T in an F-tuple. For instantiation, an NtoR-tuple is used. NtoC-tuples are used to assign codes from concept-based terminologies or classification systems that are not designed under a realist perspective.

Chapter 7
Implementations of Ontology/Terminologies and their Terminological Standards

Peter L. Elkin and Steven H. Brown

National and international standards have been developed over the last 25 years that serve to guide our generation and use of healthcare terminologies. These have been hard fought and are the result of many individuals' dedication and effort. We benefit through the use of these industry-wide agreements so that we can have consistency in today's terminology efforts. That said, current terminology efforts do not always implement best practice as we know it. This is in part because initial terminology development and dissemination is harder using formal terminologies. There is a shortage of competent terminological workers. Those who learn and can apply these

P. L. Elkin (✉)
Department of Biomedical Informatics, Jacobs School of Medicine and Biomedical Sciences, University at Buffalo, State University of New York, Buffalo, NY, USA

Internal Medicine, Jacobs School of Medicine and Biomedical Sciences, University at Buffalo, State University of New York, Buffalo, NY, USA

Surgery, Jacobs School of Medicine and Biomedical Sciences, University at Buffalo, State University of New York, Buffalo, NY, USA

Pathology and Anatomical Sciences, Jacobs School of Medicine and Biomedical Sciences, University at Buffalo, State University of New York, Buffalo, NY, USA

Psychiatry, Jacobs School of Medicine and Biomedical Sciences, University at Buffalo, State University of New York, Buffalo, NY, USA

Orthopedics, Jacobs School of Medicine and Biomedical Sciences, University at Buffalo, State University of New York, Buffalo, NY, USA
e-mail: elkinp@buffalo.edu;
http://medicine.buffalo.edu/departments/biomedical-informatics.html

S. H. Brown
Department of Veterans Affairs, Office of Health Informatics, Knowledge Based Systems, Washington, DC, USA

Department of Biomedical Informatics, Vanderbilt University, Nashville, TN, USA
e-mail: steven.brown@va.gov

P. L. Elkin (ed.), *Terminology, Ontology and their Implementations*, Health Informatics, https://doi.org/10.1007/978-3-031-11302-4_7

principles of terminological best practice will be well prepared to assist the clinical enterprise toward safer and higher quality healthcare at a lower cost.

This chapter does not discuss the standardized terminologies themselves, and it does not discuss all of the terminologically relevant standards in health informatics. However, we do provide detailed insight to several of the important standards and how they might relate to terminological quality.

You are encouraged to become involved with these terminological standardization efforts and in this way to lend your talents to those who have struggled to elevate the current terminological standards to their current level of rigor.

Questions

1. What SDO publishes TS17117? (d)

   (a) ASTM
   (b) HL7
   (c) DICOM
   (d) ISO

   ISO TC 215 publishes ISO TS 17117. This is the technical specification defining the quality indicators for healthcare terminologies. Therefore (d) is the correct answer.

2. What SDO publishes EN 12611? (b)

   (a) IHTSDO
   (b) CEN TC 251
   (c) ISO TC 215
   (d) OASIS

   CEN TC 251 is the European standards development organization and they publish EN 12611. This standard defines the categorial structures for healthcare devices. Therefore answer (b) is the correct answer.

3. The national electrical manufacturer's association is associated with which standard? (a)

   (a) DICOM
   (b) Reference Information Model
   (c) SNOMED CT
   (d) Quality indicators for HIT

   NEMA or the national electrical manufacturer's association produces standards used by the radiological community. They put out DICOM which is a standard for the representation of image data and the metadata associated with the image including clinical, transactional, and technical information. Therefore (a) is the correct answer.

4. A standard for developing models in the healthcare domain includes? (d)

   (a) HL7
   (b) SNOMED CT
   (c) OMG
   (d) All of the above

Many SDOs and specific standards define models from the healthcare domain. Conflicting standards can be useful if they lead to the resolution of unanswered questions or new and useful approaches. Here HL7 and OMG are SDOs and SNOMED CT is a terminological standard. It is not clear that these will eventually become fully coordinated. These organizations and standards create models meant to represent health-related data. This is meant to inform readers that healthcare models can be found at the core of SDOs as well as in particular terminological implementations. Therefore, answer (d) is the correct answer.

5. All of the following organizations create content for healthcare except? (c)

   (a) SNOMED CT
   (b) HL7
   (c) ISO TC 215
   (d) ASTM

   ISO TC 215 working group 3 on healthcare terminologies has as one of its principles that will not create content for health care (i.e., its own terminology). As they espoused this as a core defining principles, the ISO TC 215 WG 3 workplan does not include the generation of terminologies or terminological content. Therefore, answer (c) is the correct answer.

6. NCHS is a part of which US Government Agency? (b)

   (a) FDA
   (b) CDC
   (c) NIH
   (d) ONC

   The National Committee on Health Statistics (NCHS) is a part of the Centers for Disease Control and Prevention (CDC). Therefore, answer (b) is the correct answer.

7. Which pair(s) of standards is/are related? (d)

   (a) ASTM 2087 and ISO TS 17117
   (b) HL7 RIM and CEN 13606
   (c) ASTM CCR and HL7 CCD
   (d) a and c
   (e) a, b, and c

   ASTM 2087 was the US ANSI standard that contributed its content to ISO TS17117 and ASTM CCR was the US ANSI standard whose content was incorporated into the HL7 CDA to create the HL7 CCD. The HL7 RIM is the US standard of an overarching model for health data, and CEN 13606 is the European standard for representing electronic healthcare data. These are in some senses competitive standards representing some of the same content in different ways. Therefore, they are not complementary but competitive and were completed by different constituencies independently. Therefore, answer (d) is correct as both (a) and (c) are related standards that hold much of the same content and semantics.

8. Which standard concerns itself principally with the human–computer interaction? (c)

   (a) HL7
   (b) ASTM
   (c) CDISC
   (d) OASIS

   CDISC specifies standards for the human—computer interaction. This has taken substance around the problem of single logon, so that if you are signed on to one application your permissions can be known and where you have permissions allow you to sign on to other application maintaining your patient context (e.g., looking at data in more than one application regarding the same patient). Therefore, answer (c) is the correct answer.

9. Which standard represents methods for the transport layer standards? (a)

   (a) OASIS
   (b) HL7
   (c) CDISC
   (d) ASTM

   OASIS published electronic business XML (ebXML) which is a transport layer used to communicate terminological information. Neither HL7, CDISC, or American Society for Testing and Materials (ASTM) specify a standard for the transport layer. Therefore, the correct answer is (a).

10. Which SDO provides all of the knowledge needed for health and healthcare? (e)

    (a) HL7
    (b) ASTM
    (c) ISO TC 215
    (d) CEN TC 251
    (e) None of the above

    None of the current standards development organizations (SDO)s provide all of the knowledge needed for health and healthcare. In contrast, all of the SDOs provide some content that the other SDOs do not provide, demonstrating the strength of our intellectual community. Therefore, (e) is the correct answer.

Chapter 8
Implementations of Terminologies

Peter L. Elkin, Steven H. Brown, Stuart J. Nelson, Joan Kapusnik-Uner, Reem Mohamed, and Marjorie Rallins

P. L. Elkin (✉)
Department of Biomedical Informatics, Jacobs School of Medicine and Biomedical Sciences, University at Buffalo, State University of New York, Buffalo, NY, USA

Internal Medicine, Jacobs School of Medicine and Biomedical Sciences, University at Buffalo, State University of New York, Buffalo, NY, USA

Surgery, Jacobs School of Medicine and Biomedical Sciences, University at Buffalo, State University of New York, Buffalo, NY, USA

Pathology and Anatomical Sciences, Jacobs School of Medicine and Biomedical Sciences, University at Buffalo, State University of New York, Buffalo, NY, USA

Psychiatry, Jacobs School of Medicine and Biomedical Sciences, University at Buffalo, State University of New York, Buffalo, NY, USA

Orthopedics, Jacobs School of Medicine and Biomedical Sciences, University at Buffalo, State University of New York, Buffalo, NY, USA
e-mail: elkinp@buffalo.edu;
http://medicine.buffalo.edu/departments/biomedical-informatics.html

S. H. Brown
Department of Veterans Affairs, Vanderbilt University, Nashville, TN, USA
e-mail: steven.brown@va.gov

S. J. Nelson
Biomedical Informatics Center, George Washington University, Washington, DC, USA

J. Kapusnik-Uner
First Databank (FDB), San Bruno, CA, USA

School of Pharmacy, University of California San Francisco, San Francisco, CA, USA
e-mail: jkapusnik-uner@fdbhealth.com

R. Mohamed
First Databank (FDB), San Bruno, CA, USA

M. Rallins
Reginstrief Institute, Indianapolis, IN, USA
e-mail: mrallins@regenstrief.org

P. L. Elkin (ed.), *Terminology, Ontology and their Implementations*, Health Informatics, https://doi.org/10.1007/978-3-031-11302-4_8

For many, this is where the chapter is where the rubber meets the road in healthcare terminologies. Here, we discuss many of the individual terminologies used in health care, their history and development, their structure, use and their strengths and weaknesses. Terminology workers should be familiar with each of these terminologies and should have a sense of when to employ them in their practice.

It should be evident in your practice where tradeoffs between efficiencies and best terminological practice have been made by each SDO engaged in the creation of a health terminology. This will help the reader to recognize the strengths and weaknesses of each terminology and therefore know their limitations. Should the reader go on to create a healthcare terminology in the future, it should serve as lessons learned to understand these tradeoffs in the context of best practice of terminological development and classification.

These questions are meant to test the readers' knowledge of the terminological implementations discussed in this chapter.

Questions

1. The UMLS Knowledge sources includes? (d)

   (a) Semantic Network
   (b) Specialist Lexicon
   (c) The Metathesaurus
   (d) All of the above
   (e) b and c

   The UMLS Knowledge sources include the Metathesaurus that holds the health terminologies and their mappings to CUIs. The Semantic Network that connects concepts by their CUIs across the Metathesaurus and the Specialist Lexicon which provides software utilities, and data to support natural language processing. Therefore, (d) all of the above is the correct answer.

2. The UMLS Metathesaurus includes? (c)

   (a) One integrated terminology
   (b) A merger of multiple terminologies
   (c) A set of separate terminologies
   (d) A semantic network

   It is important to remember that the UMLS Metathesaurus does not integrate its component terminologies into one large terminology with a consistent set of content and structure. Instead, each component terminology that contributes to Metathesaurus retains its own content and hierarchies. This is a philosophical basis of the Metathesaurus. The semantic network is a separate component of the UMLS knowledge sources. Neither are the separate terminologies merged into one terminology nor are they truly integrated. Therefore, (c) is the correct answer.

3. The NLM stands for? (b)

   (a) The Natural Language Machine
   (b) The National Library of Medicine

   (c) The Natural Library of Medicine
   (d) The Nation Library of Machine Learning

   The NLM is the National Library of Medicine. Therefore, answer (b) is correct.

4. The UMLS terminologies can be found in? (c)

   (a) The Specialist Lexicon
   (b) The Semantic Network
   (c) The Metathesaurus
   (d) None of the above

   The UMLS Metathesaurus contains the specific terminologies that contribute to the UMLS. Therefore, the correct answer is (c).

5. The UMLS Semantic Network has how many semantic types? (a)

   (a) 133
   (b) 103
   (c) 163
   (d) 193

   The UMLS Semantic Network has 133 semantic types. Therefore, answer (a) is correct.

6. In the UMLS, terminological information is linked by CUIs which stands for? (c)

   (a) Contents Unique Identifiers
   (b) Contents Unified by Identifiers
   (c) Concept Unique Identifiers
   (d) Concept Unified by Identifiers

   The acronym CUIs stands for Concept Unique Identifiers. Therefore, answer (c) is correct.

7. UMLS semantic types are classified as either? (b)

   (a) Objects or classes
   (b) Entities or events
   (c) Entry or event
   (d) Entry or act

   UMLS semantic types are classified as either events or entities. Therefore, (b) is the correct answer.

8. The difference between an SUI and an AUI is? (d)

   (a) There are more SUIs than AUIs
   (b) There are more AUIs than SUIs
   (c) SUIs are unique to a string and a terminology
   (d) AUIs are unique to a string and a terminology

   Atom Unique Identifiers (AUIs) are unique to a string and a terminology, whereas String Unique Identifiers (SUIs) are unique to the string, so that if that string appears in multiple terminologies there would be more than one AUI but only one SUI. Although there are probably more AUIs than SUIs, this is not the best answer as it does not differentiate what is meant by an AUI from what is meant as an SUI. Answers (a) and (c) are incorrect. Therefore, the correct answer is (d).

9. Synonyms in the UMLS are found in which file? (b)

   (a) MRREL.RRF
   (b) MRCONSO.RRF
   (c) MRDEF.RRF
   (d) MRSTY.RRF

   Synonyms in the UMLS are distributed in and can be found in the MRCONSO.RRF file. Therefore, (b) is the correct answer.

10. The UMLS is updated? (b)

   (a) Once a year
   (b) Twice a year
   (c) Three times a year
   (d) Four times a year

   The UMLS is updated and released every 6 months; therefore, (b) is the correct answer. As the UMLS is more often used locally than in a distributed environment, it is not practical to make the rereleases too often for either the developers or the consumers of healthcare terminologies.

11. The WHO Family of Classifications include all of the following except? (c)

   (a) International Classification of Diseases (ICD)
   (b) International Classification of Function (ICF)
   (c) International Classification of Nursing Practice (ICNP)
   (d) International Classification of Health Interventions (ICHI)

   The ICNP is not a product of the WHO. The other terminologies that have the start International Classification noted above are all part of the WHO Family of Classifications. It shows that names can be deceiving as these are not trademarked across countries. Therefore, (c) is the correct answer.

12. In the United States, which version of the ICD is used to record a person's death? (d)

   (a) ICD9
   (b) ICD9-CM
   (c) ICD10-AM
   (d) ICD10

   Several years ago, the United States switched its standard for mortality coding from ICD9-CM to ICD10. We still do not know how much better the mortality data will be with the use of ICD10 as we do not have enough data to come to conclusions. Overall ICD10 is about four times the size of ICD9-CM. ICD9 as distributed by the WHO and ICD10-AM which is the Australian Modification of ICD10 are both not used as standards in the United States. Therefore, (d) is the correct answer.

13. Which version of ICD is used most commonly in research to record a patient's morbidity? (b)

    (a) ICD9
    (b) ICD9-CM
    (c) ICD10-AM
    (d) ICD10

    In the United States, the answer for morbidity coding is ICD9-CM or clinically modified. The NCHS does this modification and ICD9-CM is also used for recording diagnoses associated with the billing records from healthcare encounters and hospitalizations. Therefore, ICD9-CM I is the best answer (b).

14. ICD9-CM is maintained by? (a)

    (a) The CDC
    (b) The NLM
    (c) The WHO
    (d) The IHTSDO

    ICD9 is distributed by the WHO. In the United States, NCHS which is part of the CDC modified ICD9 to create ICD9-CM. Therefore, (a) the CDC is the correct answer.

15. Error rates in ICD9-CM code assignments are best represented by which rate? (d)

    (a) 2%
    (b) 12%
    (c) 22%
    (d) 32%

    The error rates from the healthcare literature associated with ICD9-CM coding are between 23% and 40%. Therefore, (d), 32%, is the best answer.

16. Which of the following statements are true? (d)

    (a) SNOMED CT has more concepts than ICD9-CM
    (b) ICD9-CM has more concepts than SNOMED-CT
    (c) ICD9-CM has been used in more research projects than SNOMED CT
    (d) a and c
    (e) b and c

    SNOMED CT has approximately 291,000 active concepts, whereas ICD9-CM has approximately 16,000 concepts. However, due to ICD9-CM being the standard for morbidity coding in the United States, it has been used more often for clinical care and therefore has been more available for use in research. To date, many more research projects have employed ICD9-CM than SNOMED CT. Therefore, (d) is the correct answer, as items (a) and (c) are both correct.

17. The following terminologies have a description logic basis except? (d)

    (a) SNOMED CT
    (b) ICNP
    (c) NDF-RT
    (d) LOINC

    SNOMED CT, ICNP, and NDF-RT are all based on a description logic formalism. LOINC is a pre-coordinated terminology. Therefore, (d), LOINC, is the correct answer.
18. The following terminologies have pre-coordinated concepts? (d)

    (a) LOINC
    (b) RxNorm
    (c) ICD9-CM
    (d) All of the above

    LOINC and ICD9-CM are primarily pre-coordinated terminologies. Although NDF-RT is description logic based, it still has many pre-coordinated concepts within its terminology. Therefore, the correct answer is (d) all of the above.
19. Which terminologies have been used as a reference terminology? (e)

    (a) SNOMED CT
    (b) ICF
    (c) NDF-RT
    (d) LOINC
    (e) a and c

    SNOMED CT and the NDF-RT have both been used as reference terminologies. ICF and LOINC have not been used together with an interface terminology to record data. Therefore, (e) is the correct answer.
20. SNOMED CT is maintained by the? (b)

    (a) WHO
    (b) IHTSDO
    (c) NLM
    (d) CDC

    SNOMED CT is maintained by the International Health Terminology Standards Development Organization (IHTSDO). Therefore, (b) is the correct answer.
21. The form of Compositional Expressions in SNOMED CT are governed by? (c)

    (a) Common sense
    (b) The Description Logic Handbook
    (c) The SNOMED CT style guide
    (d) The IHTSO handbook

The SNOMED CT style guide provides the rules for creating compositional expressions using SNOMED CT. This is an authoring guide that seeks to create consistency in authoring across modelers. Therefore, (c) is the correct answer.

22. In SNOMED CT, the description logic definitions are used? (d)

    (a) To serve as a formal definition for the concept
    (b) To find a concepts place in the SNOMED CT hierarchy
    (c) To find conflicts in the terminology
    (d) All of the above

    Description logic definitions have multiple purposes within a formal terminological system. In SNOMED CT, the DL holds formal definitions of each concept, allows the classifier to find the correct location(s) that the concept should be represented within the SNOMED CT hierarchical structure and can be used to find collisions or conflicts within the terminology, where two or more concepts have the same formal definitions. In cases like this either some of the definitions need to be changed or the concepts need to be conflated into a smaller number of unique concepts. Therefore, (d) is the correct answer.

23. LOINC was originally created to represent? (b)

    (a) Radiological knowledge
    (b) Laboratory knowledge
    (c) Pathological knowledge
    (d) Clinical practice knowledge

    The LOINC terminology was originally created to hold knowledge associated with laboratory test results. Therefore, (b) is the correct answer.

24. LOINC is maintained by? (e)

    (a) WHO
    (b) IHTSDO
    (c) NLM
    (d) CDC
    (e) Regenstrief Institute

    LOINC is maintained by the LOINC committee and is associated with the Regenstrief Institute at Indiana University School of Medicine. The correct answer is (e).

25. The UMLS contains? (d)

    (a) LOINC
    (b) SNOMED CT
    (c) ICD9-CM
    (d) All of the above

    LOINC, SNOMED CT, and ICD9-CM are all source vocabularies in the UMLS Metathesaurus. Therefore, (d), all of the above, is the correct answer.

26. Which of the following is/are true? (a)

    (a) NDF-RT and RxNorm have some of the same concepts
    (b) NDF-RT and RxNorm have all the same concepts
    (c) NDF-RT and RxNorm have the same hierarchical information
    (d) NDF-RT and RxNorm are both maintained by the NLM

    Although RxNorm had its start concepts associated with NDF-RT, the two languages have grown somewhat apart. The NLM maintains RxNorm while the Veterans Administration (VA) maintains NDF-RT. These two terminologies both hold clinical drug information, but the information associated with the drug does differ. Therefore, each terminology has a distinct hierarchical structure. Therefore, (a) is the correct answer.
27. Which of the following is/are true? (b)

    (a) LOINC concepts can be post-coordinated
    (b) LOINC analytes are multipart names
    (c) LOINC components are compositional
    (d) LOINC clinical concepts are limited to laboratory-related clinical findings

    LOINC analytes are multipart names. They cannot be used for post-coordination and their components are not compositional, meaning one has to use the existing codes to be conformant with the standard. The clinical concepts are not limited to the laboratory domain. In fact, there is an entire section of LOINC dedicated to general clinical care and LOINC has been chosen as the standard for the coding of sections from the clinical record. Therefore, answer (b) is correct.
28. The five-digit subdivisions were developed for? (c)

    (a) ICD0
    (b) ICD5
    (c) ICD9
    (d) ICD10

    ICD9 was the first version of the ICD series from the WHO to expand the codes to five digits (of the form XXX.XX). This helped to expand the hierarchies associated with ICD9-CM. Therefore, (c) is the correct answer.
29. SNOMED CT was formed as a merger of? (b)

    (a) ICD9-CM and LOINC
    (b) CAPs terminology effort and the NHS terminology effort
    (c) Reed codes v2 and SNOMED International
    (d) Clinical terms v3 and SNOMED II

    SNOMED CT was a merger of Clinical terms v3 from the United Kingdom's NHS's terminological efforts and the College of American Pathologists (CAP) SNOMED-RT which stood for SNOMED—Reference Terminology. LOINC and ICD9-CM were both later partially incorporated into SNOMED CT. The

Reed codes were a precursor to Clinical terms v3 as SNOMED II and SNOMED International or SNOMED III were precursors to SNOMED RT and CT. Therefore, (b) is the correct answer.

30. SNOMED CT has its headquarters in? (c)

    (a) The United States
    (b) Great Britain
    (c) Denmark
    (d) France

    The IHTSDO was established in March of 2007 and made its headquarters in Copenhagen, Denmark. In April of 2007, the IHTSDO acquired the intellectual property rights to SNOMED CT for the purpose of furthering the development, standardization, and dissemination of the health terminology. Therefore, (c), Denmark, is the correct answer.

31. OCD in RxNorm stands for? (c)

    (a) Obsessive Compulsive Disorder
    (b) Overly Crowded Directory
    (c) Obsolete Clinical Drug
    (d) Open Component Drug

    RxNorm marks obsolete clinical drugs as (OCD). Obsolescent marking includes keeping the original identifier intact and providing a pointer to any new concept that is created to represent a new form of the same drug. This can happen when perhaps a drug name stays the same but its ingredients change. Therefore, answer (c) is correct.

32. SNOMED CT's coverage rate for clinical problems using only pre-coordination is? (b)

    (a) 61.4%
    (b) 51.4%
    (c) 41.4%
    (d) 31.4%

    SNOMED CT was found to have a content coverage rate of 51.4% for clinical problems in a 2006 article. Therefore, (b) is the correct answer.

33. SNOMED CT's coverage rate for clinical problems using post-coordination is? (b)

    (a) 100%
    (b) 92.3%
    (c) 82.3%
    (d) 72.3%

    In the same study referenced in question 32, the content coverage rate of SNOMED CT for clinical problems was 92.3%. Therefore, (b) is the correct answer.

34. SNOMED CT is maintained by? (a)

    (a) IHTSDO
    (b) IMIA
    (c) NLM
    (d) CAP

    SNOMED CT is maintained by the International Health Terminology Standards Development Organization (IHTSDO). Therefore, (a) is the correct answer.

35. Which statements are true regarding SNOMED CT? (c)

    (a) SNOMED CT covers all nursing content
    (b) SNOMED CT covers all clinical drugs
    (c) SNOMED CT has incorporated lab LOINC into its hierarchies
    (d) SNOMED CT has incorporated all of ICD10 into its hierarchies

    SNOMED CT has indeed incorporated laboratory LOINC codes into its hierarchy. It does not cover all nursing content or all clinical drugs nor has it incorporated all of ICD10 into its content and hierarchies. Therefore, (c) is the correct answer.

36. The therapeutic intent hierarchy is from? (b)

    (a) SNOMED CT
    (b) NDF-RT
    (c) RxNorm
    (d) LOINC

    Only NDF-RT contains a hierarchy named therapeutic intent which contains the indications for specific clinical drugs. Therefore, (b) is the correct answer.

37. Nursing terminologies include all the following except the? (c)

    (a) ICNP
    (b) NANDA
    (c) ICHI
    (d) LOINC

    The International Classification of Healthcare Interventions is sponsored by the WHO and is not, per say, a nursing-specific terminology. LOINC has been recognized by the American Nurses Association (ANA) as a nursing terminology, as has the International Classification of Nursing Practice (ICNP) and has NANDA which contains nursing diagnoses. Therefore, (c) is the correct answer.

38. In ICNP, an attribute of focus is? (d)

    (a) Concentration
    (b) Adjustment
    (c) Focal length
    (d) Timing

In reviewing the ICNP model, we can see that timing is an attribute of focus. Hence, timing helps to refine focus in the ICNP model. Therefore, (d) is the correct answer.

39. ICNP is distributed in? (b)
    (a) Common Logic
    (b) OWL
    (c) LOINC format
    (d) SNOMED CT format

    ICNP is distributed in the Web Ontology Language (OWL). The OWL format is different than that in which Common Logic, LOINC, or SNOMED CT are distributed. Therefore, (b) is the correct answer.
40. Nursing terminologies have led the development of? (c)
    (a) Concept based terminologies
    (b) Description logics
    (c) Goal statements
    (d) Mortality coding

    The representation of goal statements has been one of the many major contributions of the nursing informatics community to healthcare terminologies. Concept-based terminologies and description logics are more general notions connected to terminologies in general and are not attributed to any one informatics community. Mortality coding predates that field of Health Informatics unless you believe that Hippocrates was the first Health Informatician. Therefore, (c) is the best answer.
41. When was CPT first published? (c)
    (a) 1956
    (b) 1960
    (c) 1966
    (d) 1976

    CPT was first published in 1966. In the 1980s, it was adopted for billing by the Centers for Medicare and Medicaid Services who pay for about 380 billion dollars a year in healthcare services. CPT is still the standard for documenting procedures in the United States.
42. How many categories exist for CPT codes? (b)
    (a) 2
    (b) 3
    (c) 4
    (d) 5

    There are three main categories for CPT. Category I codes document procedures and services. Category II codes document the results of quality-of-care measurements. For example, assessment of unhealthy alcohol use would be one such measure. Category III codes document emerging devices, procedures, and services. These help the FDA follow investigational entities and methods and are considered temporary codes.

43. How many sections are the Category I CPT codes subdivided into? (b)

    (a) 2
    (b) 6
    (c) 4
    (d) 5

    CPT codes are divided into six sections. These sections are Surgery, Anesthesiology, Radiology, "Pathology and Laboratory," Medicine, and "Evaluation and Management."

44. The assignment of a procedure or service to a specific CPT section restricts its use by specific healthcare specialties. True or False? (b)

    (a) True
    (b) False

    The assignment of context in the terminology does not restrict the use or assignment. For example, asthma can be cared for by either a pulmonologist or an allergist.

45. CPT Category III codes are permanent tracking codes used to report the supply of drugs. True or False? (b)

    (a) True
    (b) False

    These codes are temporary and used to track investigational entities. Once approved by the FDA a new permanent code would be developed.

46. What does it mean to have names at a "given level of abstraction"? (b)

    (a) It defines a level in the hierarchy
    (b) It defines relations true about all the subtypes
    (c) It defines the siblings of a term
    (d) It defines the parents of a term

47. RxNorm Book Chapter Discussion Question Notes.
48. What does it mean to have names at a "given level of abstraction"?
49. There are many levels where medications could be described. Anywhere from the lot number where the medication was produced, the manufactured product name and package size, to the ingredient or ingredients it contains, or to the class of medications to which it belongs. All of these levels could be useful at one level or another. The level chosen is one at clinical discourse is common.
50. What is the advantage of using 11-digit NDC codes?

51. Most computer systems do not recognize hyphens as part of numbers. Thus a 10-digit code, separated by hyphens is converted into 10 digits with no spaces between the numbers. In that way, a code with a form of 5-3-2 digits and a code with a form of 4-4-2 digits could be identical (and therefore not unique) without the hyphens.
52. Why do you think RxNorm was so widely adopted so readily?
53. Not only was there a recognized need (at HL7, an international standards organization) for such a product, it was simple and easily understood and explained. That it could rapidly cover so many products was an additional benefit. And that it was available at no cost made it highly acceptable.
54. What is the advantage of leaving some products out of scope of RxNorm?
55. One of the maxims of computer science is to handle exceptional problems exceptionally, while the coverage of RxNorm could handle so many products, with only a few exceptions made provided an extraordinary ability to implement the motto of "a simple idea implemented rigorously."
56. Why does RxNorm update so frequently?
57. New drugs appear on the market with amazing frequency. If RxNorm is to be used in a rapidly evolving environment, it must provide those updates quickly.
58. Does RxNorm eliminate the need for electronic health records to use a pharmacy knowledge base?
59. RxNorm does not include classes of drugs as a regular procedure. Each Pharmacy Knowledge Base has a somewhat different method of representing classes and have classes with different members. RxNorm does not include other information often useful, such as that used for drug interaction checking, pricing information, including rebates and other promotions. Having this information not in RxNorm is an advantage to the user.

Chapter 9
Terminological Systems

Peter L. Elkin and Steven H. Brown

Terminologies would not function well without terminological systems. These systems make possible the use of formal logical systems such as description logics and conceptual graphs. Without these systems maintaining consistency across large terminologies (>20,000 concepts) would be impossible.

We discuss the three main classes of terminological systems. Those systems intended to author and maintain terminologies, those systems intended to use the terminology to code clinical documentation and those systems which make secondary use of healthcare data.

P. L. Elkin (✉)
Department of Biomedical Informatics, Jacobs School of Medicine and Biomedical Sciences, University at Buffalo, State University of New York, Buffalo, NY, USA

Internal Medicine, Jacobs School of Medicine and Biomedical Sciences, University at Buffalo, State University of New York, Buffalo, NY, USA

Surgery, Jacobs School of Medicine and Biomedical Sciences, University at Buffalo, State University of New York, Buffalo, NY, USA

Pathology and Anatomical Sciences, Jacobs School of Medicine and Biomedical Sciences, University at Buffalo, State University of New York, Buffalo, NY, USA

Psychiatry, Jacobs School of Medicine and Biomedical Sciences, University at Buffalo, State University of New York, Buffalo, NY, USA

Orthopedics, Jacobs School of Medicine and Biomedical Sciences, University at Buffalo, State University of New York, Buffalo, NY, USA
e-mail: elkinp@buffalo.edu;
http://medicine.buffalo.edu/departments/biomedical-informatics.html

S. H. Brown
Department of Veterans Affairs, Office of Health Informatics, Knowledge Based Systems, Washington, DC, USA

Department of Biomedical Informatics, Vanderbilt University, Nashville, TN, USA
e-mail: steven.brown@va.gov

P. L. Elkin (ed.), *Terminology, Ontology and their Implementations*, Health Informatics, https://doi.org/10.1007/978-3-031-11302-4_9

Each of these categories holds a variety of individual implementations of terminological systems. We provide a few examples of terminological systems that have gained some prominence in the field. By reviewing these examples, we hope that the reader will gain an understanding of the types of software available in each of these categories and what has been a robust legacy of interesting work in the area of knowledge representation in health care.

To date, no commercial electronic health record (EHR) vendors have made full use of terminological systems, and hence the level of interoperability provided by these systems is lower if they had adopted a robust terminological infrastructure. As we are pushed toward interoperable health records and we increasingly are required to make secondary use of the clinical data for electronic quality and safety monitoring and reporting, we will need even more rigorous and complete terminological systems to support clinical meaning across the healthcare enterprise in the United States and eventually globally.

We have chosen not to test students on the details of individual terminological systems as we wanted to emphasize the principles associated with terminological systems rather than specific implementations themselves.

Questions

1. Terminological systems include? (d)

    (a) MetaMap
    (b) IHTSDO Workbench
    (c) Negex
    (d) All of the above

    MetaMap a natural language processor from the NLM, the IHTSDO Workbench for terminological development and maintenance and Negex an open source NLP engine with negation detection are all examples of terminological systems. Therefore, the correct answer is (d), all of the above.

2. The secondary use of clinical data? (b)

    (a) Includes all uses of clinical data
    (b) Does not include clinical uses of healthcare data
    (c) Includes natural language processing software
    (d) Does not include decision support

    The secondary use of clinical data can include many uses other than its primary use which is for the care of an individual patient and their family. It does not include all uses of clinical data. Nor does it include NLP software. Secondary uses of clinical data can drive clinical decision support so (d) is incorrect. Therefore, the best answer is (b).

3. Which correctly lists the order from oldest to newest of these terminology development platforms? (c)

    (a) Apelon TDE, IHTSDO Workbench, Protégé
    (b) Protégé, Apelon TDE, IHTSDO Workbench

(c) Apelon TDE, Protégé, IHTSDO Workbench
(d) IHTSDO Workbench, Apelon TDE, Protégé

Of the three terminology development environment in this question, the oldest is the Apelon TDE, then Protégé and the most recently developed terminological system is the IHTSDO Workbench. Therefore, answer (c) is the correct answer.

4. Which natural language processor was built by the National Library of Medicine? (a)

   (a) MetaMap
   (b) iNLP
   (c) NegEx
   (d) OpenNLP

   MetaMap was developed by the National Library of Medicine (NLM). iNLP, NegEx and OpenNLP were not developed by NLM but many were developed using funds from NLM extramural grants and contracts. Therefore, (a) is the correct answer.

5. IBM's Watson Computer employs which of the following? (c)

   (a) SNOMED CT
   (b) HL7 RIM
   (c) UIMA
   (d) ISO TS17117

   IBM's Watson computer used NLP and a set of smart weighting algorithms for N-grams derived from authoritative text in the context of the UIMA framework to compete successfully against two of the best human Jeopardy contestants. IBM hopes to leverage Watson in the healthcare domain. Therefore, answer (c) is correct.

6. Which of the following is not available through an open source license? (b)

   (a) UIMA
   (b) MedLEE
   (c) Protégé
   (d) IHTSDO Workbench

   UIMA, Protégé and the IHTSDO Workbench are all available under open source licenses. Therefore, (b) is the correct answer.

7. Which of the following system(s) employ a description logic classifier? (d)

   (a) Protégé
   (b) Apelon's TDE
   (c) IHTSDO Workbench
   (d) All of the above
   (e) Only a and c

   Protégé, Apelon's TDE and the IHTSDO Workbench all contain an instance of a description logic classifier which they employ to find collisions and to autoclassify content. Therefore, (d), all of the above, is the correct answer.

8. The “curly braces” problem in the field of CDS is? (c)

   (a) A syntax problem with formatting rule sets
   (b) A way to call out portions of the rule for which data is missing
   (c) Variables from clinical content that are not easily obtained to trigger rules
   (d) Parts of a rule set that hold codified data

   The “curly braces” problem in health informatics describes the phenomenon where Health Informaticians would build decision support rules where descriptions of variables were bracketed by curly braces. These often took the form of statements such as “If {Serum Sodium} < 125 mg/dl Then Trigger the Hyponatremia Guideline” where the ability to serve up actual lab data regarding the {Serum Sodium} requires that the lab’s label for Serum Sodium are known and used consistently across all the lab systems from which you have to obtain the data. Often these are not known and sometimes they change over time when new lab equipment is purchased which uses somewhat different measurement techniques. This difficulty in obtaining the data to feed decision support models is deemed by the “curly braces” problem. Therefore, (c) is the correct answer.

9. Terminological systems are important for? (d)

   (a) The development of ontologies
   (b) The use of ontologies for data mining
   (c) The secondary use of clinical data
   (d) All of the above

   Terminological systems are important for the development, maintenance, data mining and other secondary uses of clinical data. Therefore, answer (d), all of the above, is the correct answer.

10. The usability of terminological systems is? (e)

    (a) Important for the system to be usable by knowledge workers
    (b) Important for the system to be usable by subject matter experts
    (c) Important for the accuracy of terminological systems
    (d) Only a and b
    (e) a, b and c

    Human factors engineering and usability testing is very important for the accuracy and use of terminological systems. Most are designed to interact with patients or healthcare personnel who come to their work with the system with a given knowledgebase, experience and expectations. These perceptions are important not only to the system’s usability, but also usability problems can impact the accuracy of the system, as unusable systems predispose to errors. These inaccuracies are more common that most people think and can be a significant source of error. Formal usability testing should be part of the software development life cycle of all terminological systems development.

Chapter 10
The Future of Ontology and Terminologies

Peter L. Elkin and Barry Smith

1. Where should effort be placed to best advance the field of Ontology and Terminology?
2. What goals do you feel are most realizable given current technology?

P. L. Elkin (✉)
Department of Biomedical Informatics, Jacobs School of Medicine and Biomedical Sciences, University at Buffalo, State University of New York, Buffalo, NY, USA

Internal Medicine, Jacobs School of Medicine and Biomedical Sciences, University at Buffalo, State University of New York, Buffalo, NY, USA

Surgery, Jacobs School of Medicine and Biomedical Sciences, University at Buffalo, State University of New York, Buffalo, NY, USA

Pathology and Anatomical Sciences, Jacobs School of Medicine and Biomedical Sciences, University at Buffalo, State University of New York, Buffalo, NY, USA

Psychiatry, Jacobs School of Medicine and Biomedical Sciences, University at Buffalo, State University of New York, Buffalo, NY, USA

Orthopedics, Jacobs School of Medicine and Biomedical Sciences, University at Buffalo, State University of New York, Buffalo, NY, USA
e-mail: elkinp@buffalo.edu;
http://medicine.buffalo.edu/departments/biomedical-informatics.html

B. Smith
Department of Philosophy, University at Buffalo, Buffalo, NY, USA

Department of Biomedical Informatics, University at Buffalo, Buffalo, NY, USA
e-mail: phismith@buffalo.edu

P. L. Elkin (ed.), *Terminology, Ontology and their Implementations*, Health Informatics, https://doi.org/10.1007/978-3-031-11302-4_10

Chapter 11
Conclusions

Peter L. Elkin

The teachers' guide is meant to provide insight and answers to a set of questions associated with each chapter of the Terminology and Terminological Systems Textbook. We have crafted these questions so that in addition to assessing knowledge we can provide a different teaching perspective than is given in the textbook. Students that have an understanding of the material in this textbook will have a strong background in health terminologies and when combined with experience will prepare them for a career in Health Informatics with a concentration in Health Terminologies. The questions are a reflection of the material in each chapter and concentrate on making the reader comfortable with the concepts and language used in the field. We want the students to have an understanding of the major concepts in the discipline of health terminologies, and we want the students to understand the relationship between health terminology theory and practice and the implementations of health terminologies and terminological systems. Lastly, it is our goal that

P. L. Elkin (✉)
Department of Biomedical Informatics, Jacobs School of Medicine and Biomedical Sciences, University at Buffalo, State University of New York, Buffalo, NY, USA

Internal Medicine, Jacobs School of Medicine and Biomedical Sciences, University at Buffalo, State University of New York, Buffalo, NY, USA

Surgery, Jacobs School of Medicine and Biomedical Sciences, University at Buffalo, State University of New York, Buffalo, NY, USA

Pathology and Anatomical Sciences, Jacobs School of Medicine and Biomedical Sciences, University at Buffalo, State University of New York, Buffalo, NY, USA

Psychiatry, Jacobs School of Medicine and Biomedical Sciences, University at Buffalo, State University of New York, Buffalo, NY, USA

Orthopedics, Jacobs School of Medicine and Biomedical Sciences, University at Buffalo, State University of New York, Buffalo, NY, USA
e-mail: elkinp@buffalo.edu;
http://medicine.buffalo.edu/departments/biomedical-informatics.html

P. L. Elkin (ed.), *Terminology, Ontology and their Implementations*, Health Informatics, https://doi.org/10.1007/978-3-031-11302-4_11

students understand the relationship between the discipline of health terminologies and other disciplines within the field of Health Informatics. This will provide students whose interest and concentration are in other areas of Health Informatics with the knowledge to understand when they need to refer a matter to a Health Terminology Sub-Specialist. Together this textbook provides readers of all levels and interests with a background in Health Terminologies sufficient to accomplish their educational goals.